Management of Preterm Birth: Best Practices in Prediction, Prevention, and Treatment

Guest Editor

ALICE REEVES GOEPFERT, MD

OBSTETRICS AND GYNECOLOGY CLINICS OF NORTH AMERICA

www.obgyn.theclinics.com

Consulting Editor
WILLIAM F. RAYBURN, MD, MBA

March 2012 • Volume 39 • Number 1

SAUNDERS an imprint of ELSEVIER, Inc.

W.B. SAUNDERS COMPANY
A Division of Elsevier Inc.

Elsevier, Inc. • 1600 John F. Kennedy Blvd. • Suite 1800 • Philadelphia, PA 19103-2899

http://www.theclinics.com

OBSTETRICS AND GYNECOLOGY CLINICS OF NORTH AMERICA Volume 39, Number 1
March 2012 ISSN 0889-8545, ISBN-13: 978-1-4557-3900-4

Editor: Stephanie Donley

Obstetrics and Gynecology Clinics (ISSN 0889-8545) is published quarterly by Elsevier Inc., 360 Park Avenue South, New York, NY 10010-1710. Months of issue are March, June, September, and December. Periodicals postage paid at New York, NY, and additional mailing offices. Subscription price per year is $293.00 (US individuals), $498.00 (US institutions), $146.00 (US students), $353.00 (Canadian individuals), $628.00 (Canadian institutions), $214.00 (Canadian students), $428.00 (foreign individuals), $628.00 (foreign institutions), and $214.00 (foreign students). To receive student/ resident rate, orders must be accompanied by name of affiliated institution, date of term, and the signature of program/ residency coordinator on institution letterhead. Orders will be billed at individual rate until proof of status is received. Foreign air speed delivery is included in all *Clinics* subscription prices. All prices are subject to change without notice. POSTMASTER: Send address changes to *Obstetrics and Gynecology Clinics*, Elsevier Health Sciences Division, Subscription Customer Service, 3251 Riverport Lane, Maryland Heights, MO 63043. **Customer Service: Telephone: 1-800-654-2452 (U.S. and Canada); 314-447-8871 (outside U.S. and Canada). Fax: 314-447-8029.** E-mail: journalscustomerservice-usa@elsevier.com (for print support); journalsonlinesupport-usa@elsevier.com (for online support).

Reprints. For copies of 100 or more of articles in this publication, please contact the Commercial Reprints Department, Elsevier Inc., 360 Park Avenue South, New York, New York 10010-1710. Tel.: 212-633-3818; Fax: 212-462-1935; E-mail: reprints@elsevier.com.

Obstetrics and Gynecology Clinics of North America is also published in Spanish by McGraw-Hill Interamericana Editores S.A., P.O. Box 5-237, 06500, Mexico; in Portuguese by Reichmann and Affonso Editores, Rio de Janeiro, Brazil; and in Greek by Paschalidis Medical Publications, Athens, Greece.

Obstetrics and Gynecology Clinics of North America is covered in *MEDLINE/PubMed (Index Medicus), Excerpta Medica, Current Concepts/Clinical Medicine, Science Citation Index, BIOSIS, CINAHL,* and *ISI/BIOMED.*

Printed and bound by CPI Group (UK) Ltd, Croydon, CR0 4YY
Transferred to Digital Print 2011

GOAL STATEMENT

The goal of *Obstetrics and Gynecology Clinics of North America* is to keep practicing physicians up to date with current clinical practice in OB/GYN by providing timely articles reviewing the state of the art in patient care.

ACCREDITATION

The *Obstetrics and Gynecology Clinics of North America* is planned and implemented in accordance with the Essential Areas and Policies of the Accreditation Council for Continuing Medical Education (ACCME) through the joint sponsorship of the University of Virginia School of Medicine and Elsevier. The University of Virginia School of Medicine is accredited by the ACCME to provide continuing medical education for physicians.

The University of Virginia School of Medicine designates this enduring material activity for a maximum of 15 *AMA PRA Category 1 Credit*(s)™ for each issue, 60 credits per year. Physicians should only claim credit commensurate with the extent of their participation in the activity.

The American Medical Association has determined that physicians not licensed in the US who participate in this CME enduring material activity are eligible for a maximum of 15 *AMA PRA Category 1 Credit*(s)™ for each issue, 60 credits per year.

Credit can be earned by reading the text material, taking the CME examination online at http://www.theclinics.com/home/cme, and completing the evaluation. After taking the test, you will be required to review any and all incorrect answers. Following completion of the test and evaluation, your credit will be awarded and you may print your certificate.

FACULTY DISCLOSURE/CONFLICT OF INTEREST

The University of Virginia School of Medicine, as an ACCME accredited provider, endorses and strives to comply with the Accreditation Council for Continuing Medical Education (ACCME) Standards of Commercial Support, Commonwealth of Virginia statutes, University of Virginia policies and procedures, and associated federal and private regulations and guidelines on the need for disclosure and monitoring of proprietary and financial interests that may affect the scientific integrity and balance of content delivered in continuing medical education activities under our auspices.

The University of Virginia School of Medicine requires that all CME activities accredited through this institution be developed independently and be scientifically rigorous, balanced and objective in the presentation/discussion of its content, theories and practices.

All authors/editors participating in an accredited CME activity are expected to disclose to the readers relevant financial relationships with commercial entities occurring within the past 12 months (such as grants or research support, employee, consultant, stock holder, member of speakers bureau, etc.). The University of Virginia School of Medicine will employ appropriate mechanisms to resolve potential conflicts of interest to maintain the standards of fair and balanced education to the reader. Questions about specific strategies can be directed to the Office of Continuing Medical Education, University of Virginia School of Medicine, Charlottesville, Virginia.

The faculty and staff of the University of Virginia Office of Continuing Medical Education have no financial affiliations to disclose.

The authors/editors listed below have identified no professional or financial affiliations for themselves or their spouse/partner:

Adi Abromavici, MD; Kim Boggess, MD; Clarissa Bonanno, MD; Jessica Cantu, MD; Stephanie Donley, (Acquisitions Editor); Alice Goepfert, MD (Guest Editor); Cynthia Gyamfi-Bannerman, MD; Amanda L. Horton, MD; William Irvin, MD (Test Editor); Sheri M. Jenkins, MD; Melissa Mancuso, MD; Brian Mercer, MD; John Owen, MD, MSPH; Carla E. Ransom, MD; William F. Rayburn, MD, MBA (Consulting Editor); Alan T.N. Tita, MD, PhD; Ronald J. Wapner, MD; and Luisa Wetta, MD.

The authors/editors listed below identified the following professional or financial affiliations for themselves or their spouse/partner:

Amy P. Murtha, MD is on the Advisory Board for Watson Pharmaceuticals and is a consultant for Columbia Labs.

Disclosure of Discussion of non-FDA approved uses for pharmaceutical products and/or medical devices:

The University of Virginia School of Medicine, as an ACCME provider, requires that all faculty presenters identify and disclose any off-label uses for pharmaceutical and medical device products. The University of Virginia School of Medicine recommends that each physician fully review all the available data on new products or procedures prior to clinical use.

TO ENROLL

To enroll in the Obstetrics and Gynecology Clinics of North America Continuing Medical Education program, call customer service at 1-800-654-2452 or visit us online at www.theclinics.com/home/cme. The CME program is available to subscribers for an additional fee of $180.00

Contributors

CONSULTING EDITOR

WILLIAM F. RAYBURN, MD, MBA
Randolph Seligman Professor and Chair, Department of Obstetrics and Gynecology;
Chief of Staff, University Hospital, University of New Mexico Health Science Center,
Albuquerque, New Mexico

GUEST EDITOR

ALICE REEVES GOEPFERT, MD
Professor and Director of Education, Division of Maternal-Fetal Medicine, Department of
Obstetrics and Gynecology, University of Alabama at Birmingham, Birmingham, Alabama

AUTHORS

ADI ABRAMOVICI, MD
Clinical Instructor, Division of Maternal-Fetal Medicine, University of Alabama,
Birmingham, Alabama

KIM A. BOGGESS, MD
Professor, Department of Maternal Fetal Medicine, University of North Carolina School
of Medicine, Chapel Hill, North Carolina

CLARISSA BONANNO, MD
Assistant Clinical Professor, Division of Maternal Fetal Medicine, Department of
Obstetrics and Gynecology, Columbia University College of Physicians and Surgeons,
New York, New York

JESSICA CANTU, MD
Clinical Instructor, Division of Maternal-Fetal Medicine, University of Alabama,
Birmingham, Alabama

CYNTHIA GYAMFI-BANNERMAN, MD
Associate Professor of Obstetrics and Gynecology, Division of Maternal-Fetal Medicine,
Columbia University Medical Center, New York, New York

AMANDA L. HORTON, MD
Clinical Assistant Professor, Northshore University Health System, Department of
Maternal Fetal Medicine, Pritzker School of Medicine, University of Chicago, Evanston,
Illinois

SHERI M. JENKINS, MD
Associate Professor, Division of Maternal-Fetal Medicine, University of Alabama,
Birmingham, Alabama

MELISSA MANCUSO, MD
Division of Maternal Fetal Medicine, Department of Obstetrics and Gynecology,
University of Alabama, Birmingham, Birmingham, Alabama

BRIAN MERCER, MD
Professor of Reproductive Biology, Case Western Reserve University; and Director of Obstetrics & Maternal-Fetal Medicine, MetroHealth Medical Center, Cleveland, Ohio

AMY P. MURTHA, MD
Associate Professor, Division of Maternal-Fetal Medicine, Department of Obstetrics and Gynecology; Department of Pediatrics, Duke University Medical Center, Durham, North Carolina

JOHN OWEN, MD, MSPH
Division of Maternal Fetal Medicine, Department of Obstetrics and Gynecology, University of Alabama, Birmingham, Birmingham, Alabama

CARLA E. RANSOM, MD
Fellow, Division of Maternal-Fetal Medicine, Department of Obstetrics and Gynecology, Duke University Medical Center, Durham, North Carolina

ALAN T.N. TITA, MD, PhD
Associate Professor, Maternal and Fetal Medicine Division, UAB Department of Obstetrics & Gynecology, Women & Infants Center, Birmingham, Alabama

RONALD J. WAPNER, MD
Professor, Division of Maternal Fetal Medicine, Department of Obstetrics and Gynecology, Columbia University College of Physicians and Surgeons, New York, New York

LUISA WETTA, MD
Instructor/Fellow, Maternal and Fetal Medicine Division, UAB Department of Obstetrics & Gynecology, Women & Infants Center, Birmingham, Alabama

Contents

> Preterm birth—delivery before 37 weeks of gestation—is the second leading cause of infant mortality in the United States after congenital malformations. Spontaneous preterm birth, due to either preterm labor or preterm premature membrane rupture, encompasses approximately 75% of all preterm births, almost 400,000 births per year. Since the 1960s, different formulations of progesterone have been investigated for preterm birth prevention. This article addresses the use of progesterone for the prevention of preterm birth, including selection of candidates for progesterone, pharmacokinetics, dosing, and formulations. This article aims to provide a practical guide for using progesterone in clinical practice.

> Preterm birth (delivery at fewer than 37 weeks' gestation) is the most common cause of infant morbidity and mortality among nonanomalous infants in the United States. Increasing evidence has focused on associations between clinical infection, inflammation, and preterm birth. Maternal periodontal disease, which is associated with systemic inflammation, has been associated with preterm birth. Intervention trails for treatment of periodontal disease during pregnancy, however have not consistently shown a reduction in preterm birth rates. Despite the lack of reduction in preterm birth, oral health maintenance is an important part of preventive care and should be supported during pregnancy.

> Evidence supports the concept that cervical insufficiency is but 1 component of the larger and more complex preterm birth syndrome. Premature cervical ripening provides strong evidence that parturition has begun and is the result of multiple interrelated pathways and

inciting factors. Ultrasonographic screening of the cervix and treatment with cerclage for cervical shortening in the midtrimester is reserved for women with prior spontaneous preterm birth. Although cerclage benefit for short cervix <25 mm is inversely proportional to the length, it is appropriate to offer cerclage to women with cervical length <25 mm, and particularly those with a coexistent U-shaped funnel.

The focus of this article is a description of the epidemiology and management of late preterm pregnancy. Late preterm birth results from spontaneous, indicated, and sometimes elective indications. The burden of prematurity can be decreased if elective late preterm delivery is eliminated. Certain conditions absolutely warrant late preterm delivery; however, the clinician should weigh the risks of iatrogenic prematurity with the benefits of delivery for maternal or fetal indication when considering intervention for this cohort.

Even with recently declining rates, preterm birth remains a critical public health problem. Administration of antenatal corticosteroids to improve outcomes after preterm birth is one of the most important interventions in obstetrics. This article summarizes the evidence for antenatal corticosteroid efficacy and safety. Although antenatal corticosteroids are effective for singleton pregnancies at risk for preterm birth between 26 and 34 weeks' gestation, questions remain regarding the utility in specific cases such as multiple gestations, very early preterm gestations, and pregnancies complicated by intrauterine growth restriction. Uncertainty also remains about length of corticosteroid effectiveness and need for repeat or rescue courses.

A significant fraction of preterm birth results from subclinical intrauterine infection. Antimicrobial treatment during conservative management of preterm labor and premature rupture of the membranes (PROM) remote from term could treat subclinical decidual colonization. There are data supporting adjunctive antibiotic treatment during conservative management of PROM remote from term, including broad-spectrum agents. There is no consistent evidence that antibiotic treatment in the setting of preterm labor with intact membranes prolongs pregnancy or improves newborn outcomes; there is some evidence of risk. Antibiotic treatment for pregnancy prolongation should not be offered in the setting of preterm labor with intact membranes.

> Preterm birth is the leading cause of perinatal morbidity and mortality and leads to significant health care costs annually. The decision as to which tocolytic should be utilized as the first-line agent for a patient is based on multiple factors, including gestational age, the patient's medical history, common and severe side effects, and a patient's response to therapy. This summary describes the most commonly used tocolytics, their mechanisms of action, side effects, and clinical data regarding their efficacy.

> The frequency of early term births varies by patient, provider, and system characteristics. Early term deliveries in the absence of maternal or fetal indications are associated with suboptimal neonatal outcomes without evidence of maternal benefit. Demonstrated fetal lung maturity before early term birth reduced the risk of respiratory and other morbidities, but not to low levels seen at 39-40 weeks. Sometimes the risk benefit ratio of early deliveries is unclear- provider and patient's desires should direct care. Interventions that include administrative support, review of indications, and feedback to providers can dramatically reduce the frequency of early term births over time.

THE CLINICS ARE NOW AVAILABLE ONLINE!
Access your subscription at:
www.theclinics.com

Foreword

Management Strategies to Prevent Preterm Birth

We have not focused on an issue in the *Obstetrics and Gynecology Clinics of North America* about preventing preterm delivery in several years. Many advances have received attention in the past decade, so we wish to provide an important update on "Management Strategies Prevent Preterm Birth." While numerous management methods have incorporated such diagnostic evaluations as cervical length measurements and the presence or absence of fetal fibronectin, the incidence of preterm birth has changed little over the past 40 years. Uncertainty continues about the best strategies for managing preterm labor.

Infant mortality and a wide variety of morbidities, largely due to organ system immaturity, are significant among infants born very prematurely. Because of tremendous advances in the perinatal and neonatal care, increasing survival of immature infants has prompted continued reassessments about the lower limit of fetal maturation that is compatible with extrauterine life and also long-term sequelae such as neurodevelopmental disability.

Deliveries of late preterm infants in the late preterm period contribute to the increasing morbidity and costs in newborn care. These infants account for approximately 75% of all preterm births, and they constitute an increasing proportion of all singleton preterm births in the United States. As such, late preterm birth is receiving more attention in optimizing obstetrical decision-making.

Less than half of all preterm births are preceded by spontaneous labor alone. Reasons for spontaneous preterm labor and birth are multiple. Interacting comorbidities (eg, genital tract infection and periodontal disease) are described and questioned in this issue. These antecedents and contributing conditions are essential to consider, since they confound efforts to prevent and manage pregnancies at risk of preterm delivery. Approximately one-third follow preterm rupture of membranes, while one-fourth are indicated or mandated. Much of the increase in preterm deliveries in the United States is explained by rising numbers of indicated births in singleton gestations.

While prevention of preterm birth remains elusive, this issue addresses many strategies that may be achievable in select populations. The authors cite several meta-analyses to help clarify conflicting results surrounding prophylactic therapies, such as maternal progesterone and cervical cerclage. In the absence of maternal or fetal indications necessitating pregnancy intervention, management strategies described in this issue are intended to forestall preterm birth. Women identified as being at risk for preterm birth or who present with signs and symptoms of impending preterm delivery are often candidates for such medical interventions as antenatal corticosteroids and antibiotics that are intended to improve neonatal outcomes.

Obstet Gynecol Clin N Am 39 (2012) xi–xii
doi:10.1016/j.ogc.2012.02.002
0889-8545/12/$ – see front matter © 2012 Elsevier Inc. All rights reserved.

obgyn.theclinics.com

Management decisions are greatly influenced by accurate gestational dating. For well-dated pregnancies less than 34 weeks with no mandate for delivery, close observation with monitoring of uterine contractions and fetal heart rate patterns is appropriate, along with periodic cervical examinations to search for any change. For women not in advanced labor, many practitioners believe it is appropriate to prescribe intravenous magnesium sulfate initially as an attempt to inhibit contractions and potentially provide neonatal neuroprotection. The mother-to-be is also customarily given corticosteroid therapy before 34 weeks and group B streptococcal antibiotics prophylaxis at any preterm age.

Information in this special issue represents the opinions of qualified experts in maternal fetal medicine. Their contributions in providing thoughtful and balanced approaches to designing management guidelines are noteworthy. Their input is particularly important in addressing patient's and family's preconceived impressions and in providing certain practical educational materials to both the practicing obstetrician and our valued patients.

William F. Rayburn, MD, MBA
Department of Obstetrics and Gynecology
University of New Mexico School of Medicine
MSC10 5580; 1 University of New Mexico
Albuquerque, NM 87131-0001, USA

E-mail address:
wrayburn@salud.unm.edu

Preface

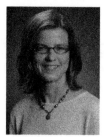

Alice Reeves Goepfert, MD
Guest Editor

Preterm birth, or delivery prior to 37 weeks' gestation, continues to be a major public health concern in the United States and is the leading cause of infant mortality excluding congenital malformations. The annual health care costs for the care of infants born preterm are substantial. However, for the first time in decades, the preterm birth rate in the United States has reached a plateau and begun to decline slightly, currently accounting for just over 12% of the 4 million births annually in the country. Fortunately, with increased public awareness to this plight of women and infants as well as funding for research and attention to outcomes by the federal government and private agencies, the busy clinician now has more effective options than ever before for screening, prevention, and treatment of women at risk for preterm birth.

In this edition of *Obstetrics and Gynecology Clinics of North America*, selected experts have been invited to review screening and prevention strategies as well as management options once preterm labor or preterm premature rupture of membranes (PROM) is diagnosed. These authors discuss the most current and relevant evidence and suggest strategies for preterm birth management based on that evidence. Importantly, the authors in this edition have not only been involved in cutting edge research in the field of preterm birth but also have busy clinical practices; they can offer therefore a practical approach to those of us struggling to determine the best options for our patients.

Drs Carla Ransom and Amy Murtha discuss the hot topic of progesterone for the prevention of preterm birth. New clinical studies on this preventive therapy are being published on a regular basis and will continue to afford healthy debate regarding the best practices. Drs Melissa Mancuso and John Owen review transvaginal ultrasound for cervical length in high-risk women and prevention strategies using cervical cerclage in the setting of a short cervix. With the recent multicenter study published by Hassan and colleagues,[1] the debate heats up regarding the efficiency of proceeding with routine screening by transvaginal ultrasound for cervical length in *low-risk women* and treatment with vaginal progesterone versus the need for additional research; clinicians are encouraged to pay attention to further discussion on this subject from leaders in the field. Although the initial excitement regarding treatment of maternal periodontal disease for the prevention of preterm birth has not been

Obstet Gynecol Clin N Am 39 (2012) xiii–xv
doi:10.1016/j.ogc.2012.02.001
0889-8545/12/$ – see front matter © 2012 Elsevier Inc. All rights reserved.

obgyn.theclinics.com

supported by several larger randomized controlled trials done in this country, Drs Amanda Horton and Kim Boggess review the evidence on this subject; clinicians are recommended to encourage oral health maintenance for maternal general health benefit.

Antenatal corticosteroids continue to be an important component of the management of women at risk for preterm birth and have resulted in improved neonatal outcome; Drs Clarissa Bonanno and Ronald Wapner discuss the history behind this treatment strategy, efficacy in special populations, choice of agent, and timing of administration. Dr Brian Mercer reviews the use of antibiotics in the management of PROM and preterm labor and presents a new meta-analysis that supports aggressive, broad-spectrum treatment for improved latency and decreased morbidity in the setting of conservative management of PROM. Drs Adi Abramovici, Jessica Cantu, and Sheri Jenkins review the use of tocolytic therapy for acute preterm labor. Magnesium sulfate for neuroprotection before anticipated preterm birth is also discussed in their article; we have adopted this strategy at our own center based on our assessment of the best available evidence. Clinicians are encouraged to review recent publications on this subject,[2,3] as well as ACOG Committee Opinion No. 455[4] and a recently published SMFM debate[5,6] to assist in their own decisions regarding use of this preventive therapy.

A component of the observed decrease in preterm births in the United States has been attributed to more conservative approaches to the delivery of late preterm births. Recommendations from a recent workshop on appropriate late preterm and early term births, cosponsored by the SMFM and NICHD, have recently been published.[7] Dr Cynthia Gyamfi-Bannerman reviews management dilemmas for these late preterm births. In addition, Drs Luisa Wetta and Alan Tita discuss considerations in management of early term births.

My hope is that this issue of *Obstetrics and Gynecology Clinics* will assist clinicians in choosing the best available options for the management of their patients at risk for preterm birth. In addition, as we continue to focus our efforts on maximizing patient safety, improving quality of care, and monitoring our patient outcomes, I hope these articles will provide guidance for improved care of women and infants.

Thank you to Elsevier for the opportunity to participate as guest editor for this issue and to Stephanie Donley, editor of *Clinics*, for her patience and persistence in making it a reality.

Alice Reeves Goepfert, MD
Division of Maternal-Fetal Medicine
Department of Obstetrics and Gynecology
University of Alabama at Birmingham
176F 10270 North, Women & Infants Center
619 19th Street South
Birmingham, AL 35249-7333, USA

E-mail address:
aliceg@uab.edu

REFERENCES

1. Hassan SS, Romero R, Vidyadhari D, et al, for the PREGNANT Trial. Vaginal progesterone reduces the rate of preterm birth in women with a sonographic short cervix: a multicenter, randomized, double-blind, placebo-controlled trial. Ultrasound Obstet Gynecol 2011;38:18–31.
2. Rouse DJ. Magnesium sulfate for the prevention of cerebral palsy. Am J Obstet Gynecol 2009;200(6):610–2.

3. Rouse DJ, Hirtz DG, Thom E, et al, Roberts JM for the Eunice Kennedy Shriver NICHD MFMU Network. A randomized, controlled trial of magnesium sulfate for the prevention of cerebral palsy. N Engl J Med 2008;359:895–905.
4. American College of Obstetricians and Gynecologists Committee on Obstetric Practice; Society for Maternal-Fetal Medicine. Committee Opinion No. 455: Magnesium sulfate before anticipated preterm birth for neuroprotection. Obstet Gynecol 2010; 115(3):669–71.
5. Rouse DJ. Magnesium sulfate for fetal neuroprotection. Am J Obstet Gynecol 2011; 205(4):296–7.
6. Sibai BM. Magnesium sulfate for neuroprotection in patients at risk for early delivery: not yet. Am J Obstet Gynecol 2011;205(4):296–7.
7. Spong CY, Mercer BM, D'Alton M, et al. Timing of indicated late-preterm and early-term birth. Obstet Gynecol 2011;118:323–33.

Progesterone for Preterm Birth Prevention

Carla E. Ransom, MD[a],*, Amy P. Murtha, MD[a,b]

KEYWORDS

- Progesterone • Progestin • Preterm birth • Prematurity
- 17α-Hydroxyprogesterone caproate

Preterm birth, defined as delivery before 37 weeks of gestation, is the second leading cause of infant mortality in the United States after congenital malformations.[1] Spontaneous preterm birth, due to either preterm labor or preterm premature rupture of membranes (PPROM), encompasses approximately 75% of all cases of preterm birth, almost 400,000 births per year.[2] Since the 1960s, different formulations of progesterone have been investigated for their role in preterm birth prevention. This article discusses the use of progesterone for the prevention of preterm birth, including selection of candidates for progesterone, pharmacokinetics, dosing, and formulations. The goal of this article is to provide a practical guide for using progesterone in clinical practice.

The incidence of preterm delivery in the United States exceeds 12% of all births, with rates of almost 18% in the non-Hispanic black population.[2] Although preterm births appear to have plateaued over the past 3 years,[3] they still remain a major public health problem. Among survivors, the prevalence of both short- and long-term morbidities, including respiratory disease, neurodevelopmental problems, and gastrointestinal disease, is estimated to be as high as 60%.[4]

COST OF PREMATURITY

Preterm birth takes a major toll on the economy. Estimates from the National Center for Health Statistics in the United States from 2005 suggest that the total national cost for the care of premature infants was in excess of $26.2 billion annually, with an average cost of care for both inpatient and outpatient services for a premature infant that was 10 times greater than for an infant born at term ($32,325 vs $3325).[5] Not

Dr Murtha attended an advisory committee meeting for Watson Pharmaceuticals and now serves as a consultant to Columbia Laboratories. Dr Murtha has attended an advisory committee meeting for Ther Rx.

[a] Division of Maternal-Fetal Medicine, Department of Obstetrics and Gynecology, Duke University Medical Center, Erwin Road, Durham, NC 27705, USA
[b] Department of Pediatrics, Duke University Medical Center, Erwin Road, Durham, NC 27705, USA
* Corresponding author.
E-mail address: carla.ransom@duke.edu

Obstet Gynecol Clin N Am 39 (2012) 1–16
doi:10.1016/j.ogc.2011.12.004
0889-8545/12/$ – see front matter © 2012 Elsevier Inc. All rights reserved.

surprisingly, the cost of care increases for infants of lower birth weight, estimated to be $140,000 if the birth weight is less than 1000 grams. Infants who suffer severe disability have long-term care costs estimated to be more than $100,000 and the cost of lifetime custodial care has been estimated to reach $450,000.[6] Further, the impact of a preterm birth on the long-term health of the individual is only beginning to be understood. It is becoming clear that, even if preterm infants surpass immediate obstacles, their overall long-term health is diminished. A recent study in Norway by Swamy and colleagues found diminished long-term survival and reproduction rates among individuals born prematurely between 1967 and 1988.[7]

PRETERM BIRTH WORLDWIDE

The problem of preterm birth spans many continents and ethnicities. In 2005, there were an estimated 12.9 million preterm births, representing almost 10% of total births worldwide.[8] By far, Africa and Asia carry the greatest burden of disease, with 11 million (85%) of these preterm births.[8] The lowest rate of preterm birth is in Europe (6.2%) while the rate in Latin America and the Caribbean is estimated to be 6.9%.[8] In the United States, the rate of preterm birth for 2009 was 12.2%.[3] This represents a third year of declining rates of preterm birth. The rate is somewhat better in Canada, but is rising in prevalence from 6.3% of live births in the 1980s to 7.6% of live births in 2000.[9] In Australia, birth before 37 weeks of gestation occurred in 7% of pregnancies within Australia during 2002, with 2.6% of all births occurring before 34 weeks of gestation. Although this represents only a small proportion of total births within Australia, it accounts for almost 70% of the total perinatal mortality.[10]

ETIOLOGY OF PRETERM BIRTH

Preterm birth is multifactorial in origin, but can broadly be divided into three basic etiologies: indicated, preterm labor (PTL), and PPROM. Indicated (iatrogenic) preterm birth, from such causes as maternal medical conditions, accounts for 25% of premature deliveries in the United States.[11] The remaining 75% accounts for spontaneous preterm birth, of which 50% is thought to be from preterm labor and 25% from PPROM. Further discussion on the etiology of preterm birth is beyond the scope of this article. However, progesterone targets the 75% of women with a history of spontaneous preterm birth.

ROLE OF PROGESTERONE IN PREGNANCY

There are many theories attempting to explain why progesterone may work to prevent preterm labor. In early pregnancy, progesterone produced by the corpus luteum is vital to pregnancy maintenance.[12] Later in gestation, the role of progesterone in humans is much less clear. Progesterone antagonists are known to stimulate labor in an animal model.[13] Several mechanisms have been proposed to address how progesterone may prevent the onset of preterm labor.

Progesterone is thought to enhance quiescence of the uterus by inhibiting uterine contractions.[14] This was initially proposed as a see-saw theory in which high levels of progesterone prevent contractions and low levels promote contractions.[15] In many animals, labor is preceded by a systemic decrease in levels of progesterone. Humans do not show this biochemical change. However, there are many biochemical changes in the uterus that are thought to lead to a "functional progesterone withdrawal."[16] Indeed, this functional withdrawal of progesterone may be related to the decreasing ability of the progesterone receptor to regulate genes that lead to uterine quiescence. It has been shown that the progesterone receptor antagonizes nuclear factor-κ-β

activation of cyclooxygenase-2 (COX-2)–induced contractility in the uterus.[17] Condon demonstrated a decline in levels of progesterone receptor coactivators in the pregnant uterus at term, which may again lead to a functional progesterone withdrawal, making the uterus more contractile while not altering the levels of circulating progesterone.[18]

Progesterone may also act at the level of the cervix. In rats, the addition of progesterone decreased levels of inducible nitric oxide synthase (iNOS) and COX-2, which are associated with cervical ripening.[19] Progestational agents have been found to modulate gene expression in the cervix, both in the presence and absence of inflammation, postulating another mechanism by which progesterone may prevent preterm births.[20] Degradation of type I collagen in the dilated cervix in labor was stimulated by the addition of physiologic concentrations of 17β-estradiol. This process was blocked by the addition of progesterone.[21,22] Basal and interleukin-1 (IL-1)–induced IL-8 production in rabbit uterine cervical fibroblasts is down-regulated by progesterone at the transcriptional level.[21,22]

The maternal immune response is another area of research. Studies have found that giving 17α-hydroxyprogesterone caproate (17-OHP-C) suppresses the maternal immune response. In patients who received exogenous 17-OHP-C, lipoteichoic acid (LTA)- or lipopolysaccharide (LPS)-stimulated induction of IL-6 was significantly decreased compared with controls.[23] The addition of exogenous progesterone has been shown in vitro to protect fetal chorion and human decidua cells from induced cell death.[24] It has been shown that the addition of progestin to term decidua cells diminishes production of IL-11, a cytokine known to enhance production of prostaglandins.[25]

Lastly, there may be autocrine and paracrine effects. Research suggests a role for placental corticotropin-releasing hormone (CRH) in the timing and initiation of labor. Rising levels of CRH are noted to precede the onset of both term and preterm labor in humans, acting as a "placental clock" to control the timing of parturition.[26] Cortisol and progesterone have competing effects on the pregnant uterus, with cortisol increasing prostaglandin production and progesterone preventing it.[27] Other studies have investigated the rising fetal cortisol levels at the end of gestation and show CRH and adrenocorticotropic hormone (ACTH) both work to down-regulate progesterone, suggesting an autocrine and paracrine effect in the initiation of human labor.[28,29]

PROGESTERONE FOR THE PREVENTION OF PRETERM BIRTH

Progestins have been investigated for the prevention of preterm birth in several different groups of women. The following subsections discuss the use of progestins for the indications of prior preterm birth, PPROM, multiple gestation, and short cervix. A summary of the major recent randomized controlled trials (RCTs) on the subject is provided in **Table 1**. Indications for use, schedule, and formulations are discussed.

Singleton Gestation with a History of Prior Preterm Birth

Research into the use of progesterone for the prevention of preterm birth dates back to the 1960s, when the first trials for its use in women with habitual abortion were published.[30] There are several published RCTs investigating this question in singleton gestation. In 1975, Johnson conducted a trial on 43 women with a history of two prior spontaneous abortions or prior preterm birth before 36 weeks of gestation who were randomized to weekly intramuscular (IM) 17-OHP-C versus placebo from "booking" until 24 weeks of gestation. He found a reduction of preterm delivery rate from 41% in the placebo group compared to 14% in the 17-OHP-C group (relative risk [RR] 0.35, 95% CI 0.11–1.11).[31] A resurgence of interest in progesterone occurred in 2003, with

Table 1
Recent randomized trials of progesterone

Author	Date, Site	Subjects	Primary Outcome	Intervention	Results
da Fonseca et al[33]	2003, Brazil	157 women at "high risk" for preterm birth	Preterm birth <37 weeks	Intravaginal progesterone (100 mg) or placebo, 24–28 weeks	RR 0.49 (95% CI 0.25–0.96)
Meis et al[32]	2003, USA	463 women with prior spontaneous PTB	Preterm birth <37 weeks	17-hydroxy-progesterone caproate (250 mg weekly) or placebo, 16–20 to 36 weeks	RR 0.66 (95% CI 0.54–0.81)
O'Brien et al[34]	2007, Multinational	659 women with prior SPTB	Preterm birth <32 weeks	Daily vaginal progesterone gel (90 mg) or placebo	RR 1.08 (95% CI 0.76–1.52)
Fonseca et al[46]	2007, UK, Brazil, Greece	250 women with cervical length ≤15 mm	Preterm birth <34 weeks	Nightly intravaginal pessary (200 mg micronized progesterone) or placebo, 24–33 + 6 weeks	RR 0.56 (95% CI 0.36–0.86)
Rouse et al[39]	2007, USA	661 twin pregnancies	Composite of delivery or death prior to 35 weeks'	Weekly IM injection of 250 mg 17-hydroxy-progesterone caproate or placebo (castor oil) from 16 to 20 + 3 weeks until 34 completed weeks	RR 1.1 (95% CI 0.9–1.3)
Hassan et al[47]	2011, USA	458 singleton pregnancies	Preterm birth before 33 weeks	Daily vaginal progesterone gel or placebo from 20 to 23 6/7 until 36 6/7 weeks	RR 0.55 (95% CI 0.33–0.92)

the publication of two trials. Meis and colleagues[32] published a multicenter trial involving 463 women with a history of prior spontaneous preterm birth who were randomized to 17-OHP-C versus placebo at a 2:1 ratio. His findings of at 36.3% rate of preterm (<37 weeks) delivery in the 17-OHP-C group versus 54.9% in the placebo group led many practitioners to adopt the use of 17-OHP-C into clinical practice (RR 0.54, 95% CI 0.54–0.81). He also found lower need for supplemental oxygen with no increase in rates of congenital anomalies. Concurrently, de Fonseca and colleagues[33] published an RCT of 157 women at high risk for preterm delivery given a history of prior spontaneous preterm birth, prophylactic cerclage, or uterine malformation and administered a vaginal progesterone suppository (100 mg) or placebo to be applied nightly from 24 to 34 weeks. This study found a 13.8% rate of preterm births of less than 37 weeks in the progesterone group compared to 28.5% in the placebo group and a 2.8% rate of preterm births of less than 34 weeks in the progesterone group compared to 18.6% in the placebo group.[33] More recently, in 2007, O'Brien and coworkers conducted an RCT investigating the use of progesterone vaginal gel (Prochieve 8%/Crinone 8% containing 90 mg progesterone gel) to reduce the recurrence of preterm birth in a group of 659 women with a history of prior spontaneous preterm birth. They found no difference in the rates of preterm birth (RR 1.08, 95% CI 0.76–1.52).[34] The discrepancies between the results of these trials may be confusing. The O'Brien trial had a preterm delivery rate in the placebo group of 40%, much higher than the rate of 28% seen in the da Fonseca trial. These trials enrolled different groups of women, with the O'Brien trial focusing on women with prior preterm birth and the da Fonseca trial having more broad inclusion criteria of women at risk for preterm delivery, such as those requiring cerclage or those with uterine anomalies. It is possible that in the da Fonseca trial, there is a subset of women who benefit most from vaginal progesterone that was just not seen in the select group studied by O'Brien and colleagues. The studies also used different doses and formulations of progesterone.

PPROM

One study[35] looked into the question of whether women with PPROM would benefit from weekly progesterone. In this study of 69 women, no differences were found in time of randomization to delivery, mode of delivery, and neonatal outcome of morbidity or mortality. At this time, there is no role for progesterone to extend gestation in women with PPROM out of a clinical trial setting.

Multiple Gestations

Women with multiple gestations are at high risk for preterm delivery. However, the etiology of preterm delivery in multiples is more complex than for singletons, with uterine stretch playing a larger role. Several studies have investigated the role of progesterone in this special population. There are four RCTs investigating the use of progesterone in twins[36–39] for a total of 1273 women and two in triplets[40, 41] for a total of 190 women. None of these investigators were able to find a difference in the rate of preterm birth or neonatal morbidity or mortality with the addition of either intramuscular 17-OHP-C[36,37,39–41] or vaginal progesterone (Crinone, 90 mg vaginal progesterone gel).[38] It is unclear whether progesterone simply does not work in this group of women or if the optimal route and dose of progesterone in women with multiple gestations have yet to be found.

Impact of Cervical Length

A short cervical length on second trimester ultrasound is among the best methods to predict spontaneous preterm birth,[42] while the most important historical risk factor is a history of prior preterm birth.[43] Given the high-risk nature of this population, several authors have looked at progesterone in women with a short cervix with or without a history of preterm birth.

In a secondary analysis of an RCT of vaginal progesterone gel (Prochieve 8%/Crinone 8% containing 90 mg progesterone gel) for the prevention of preterm birth in women with a history of preterm birth,[44] women with a cervical length of less than 28 mm at enrollment had a significantly lower rate of preterm birth at 32 weeks or less if they received progesterone versus placebo (0% vs 29.6%, $P = .014$). In addition, progesterone offered a neonatal benefit, with fewer admissions into the neonatal intensive care unit (NICU; 15.8% vs 51.9%), shorter NICU stays (1.1 vs 16.5 days, $P = .013$), and a trend toward a decreased rate of neonatal respiratory distress syndrome (5.3% vs 29.6%, $P = .060$). In their secondary analysis from this trial, O'Brien and colleagues[45] found that vaginal progesterone (Prochieve 8% containing 90 mg progesterone gel) appeared to slow the rate of cervical shortening on women with prior spontaneous preterm birth.

Another RCT of vaginal progesterone (200-mg capsules of micronized progesterone) in women with a short cervix (<15 mm) at 22 weeks of gestation[46] showed decreased rates of preterm birth less than 34 weeks of gestation (19.2% vs 34.4%, RR 0.56) with a nonsignificant trend toward lower neonatal morbidity.

The most recent trial on the use of progesterone in women with a sonographically short cervix[47] showed that in women with a cervical length between 10 and 20 mm detected between 19 and 23 6/7 weeks, the use of vaginal progesterone gel (Crinone 8%/Prochieve 8% containing 90 mg progesterone gel) resulted in a lower rate of preterm birth before 33 weeks compared to those who received placebo (8.9% vs 16.1%, $P = .02$), for an overall 45% reduction in the rate of preterm birth before 33 weeks. This study also demonstrated a lower risk of several neonatal morbidities, including respiratory distress syndrome (3.0% vs 7.6%, $P = .03$), any neonatal morbidity or mortality event (7.7% vs 13.5%, $P = .04$), and birth weight less than 1500 g (6.4% vs 13.6%, $P = .01$).

Historically, cerclage may be offered to women with a sonographically identified short cervix. It has been shown to reduce the incidence of recurrent preterm birth in the high-risk cohort of women with prior spontaneous preterm birth and short cervix (<25 mm).[48] There are few trials directly comparing the efficacy of cerclage versus progesterone. Keeler and colleagues[49] attempted to answer this question in 2009 with an RCT of 79 patients with cervical length less than or equal to 25 mm who were randomized to either cerclage or weekly 17-OHP-C. There was no difference in the primary outcome of delivery less than 35 weeks in the two groups. Of note, there was a very high rate of preterm delivery in both groups, with more than 50% delivering at less than 37 weeks. Given the small sample size and negative results, there are no good data currently comparing cerclage and progesterone. In a similar question, Berghella and coworkers[50] asked whether the addition of 17-OHP-C in women with cerclage offered additional benefit and found no additional reduction in the rate of preterm birth by adding weekly 17-OHP-C for women with cerclage placed. However, in women who did not receive cerclage, 17-OHP-C reduced previable birth and perinatal mortality.

There are scant data in women with multiple gestations who are also found to have a short cervix, although this group has more confounding given the high rate and differing etiology of preterm birth in multiples. Given that, Durnwald and colleagues[51] demonstrated in a secondary analysis that women with cervical length less than 25% had higher rates of preterm birth (55.8 vs 36.9%, $P = .02$). Weekly 17-OHP-C offered no protection against preterm birth in this population. In 2007, Facchinetti and coworkers[52] found that in women admitted with preterm labor, progesterone administration attenuated the rate of cervical shortening and resulted in lower rates of preterm delivery.

In summary, the use of progesterone for the prevention of preterm birth in women with singleton gestation and a sonographically identified short cervix can be considered. The data examining the addition of progestins to women with cerclage are limited; although the limited studies published to date showed no clear benefit, future research is needed to clarify this question. Whether there is a difference between vaginal progesterone and intramuscular 17-OHP-C in this group of women is also unclear.

Candidates for Progesterone Therapy

Current guidelines state that women with a history of prior spontaneous preterm birth, defined as delivery between 20/0 and 36/6 weeks gestation due to either spontaneous preterm labor or PPROM, be offered progestin therapy.[53] Progestin has been shown to be effective in women with a history of spontaneous preterm birth as early as 20 weeks of gestation.[54] Progestin supplementation in women with a short cervix can be considered, although at this time there are no clear guidelines for its use. There are no data to support the use of progestin therapy in women with multiple gestation, women with PPROM, women with preterm labor, or women with a positive fetal fibronectin. Use in these groups should be restricted to clinical trials.

Administration of Progesterone

Three main formulations of progestins have been studied: oral, intramuscular, and vaginal. The oral and vaginal preparations are natural progesterone while the intramuscular drug 17-OHP-C is synthetic.

The interest in using oral progesterone for the prevention of preterm birth has been investigated in two clinical trials. In 2009, Rai and colleagues[55] conducted a randomized, double-blind, placebo-controlled trial of 150 women with at least one preterm birth who received 100 mg of oral micronized progesterone (OMP) or placebo twice a day from recruitment (18–24 weeks) until 36 weeks or delivery. This study found a reduction in preterm birth in the OMP group compared to controls (39.2% vs 59.5%, $P = .0002$). There was also a reduced risk of NICU admission, low birth weight, and duration of NICU stay. In 2011, Glover and coworkers[56] published a pilot study of 33 women of women with prior spontaneous preterm birth and randomized them to either daily oral micronized progesterone (400 mg) or placebo from 16 to 34 weeks of gestation. They did not find a difference in the primary study outcome of spontaneous preterm birth. However, there was a trend toward a reduction in recurrent spontaneous preterm birth and an increase in the maternal serum progesterone in the group of women receiving progesterone.

There are several trials investigating vaginal progesterone.[10,34,57] Authors favoring this formulation point to its natural formulation and higher endometrial concentration than via intramuscular administration, with a 14 times greater increase in the ratio of endometrial to serum concentration after vaginal dosing.[58–60]

There are also several trials utilizing 17-OHP-C[61–63] for pregnancy support in the first trimester. Authors favoring this approach point to positive early trials with its use.[32] Currently, intramuscular 17-OHP-C (Makena) is the only US Food and Drug

Administration (FDA)-approved formulation of progestin with the indication of prevention of preterm birth.

Take home point: There are insufficient data on the optimal route of progesterone administration. Given a paucity of trials, use of oral progesterone for the prevention of preterm birth should be restricted to clinical trials. There are positive[32,33] and negative trials[34] involving vaginal progesterone[33,34] and intramuscular 17-OHP-C.[32] Both can be considered for use. Although Makena is the only FDA-approved formulation of 17-OHP-C with an indication for preterm birth prevention, there is significant controversy surrounding the cost of the FDA-approved product.[64]

Timing of Initiation and Cessation of Progesterone

The optimal timing for initiation of progesterone treatment has been investigated.[65,66] Most trials initiate progestin between 16/0 and 20/6 weeks of gestation. Gonzalez-Quintero and colleagues[65] and How and colleagues[66] have both shown no difference in the efficacy of 17-OHP-C when initiated between 16 and 20.9 weeks or 21 and 26.9 weeks regardless of the number of prior preterm deliveries. Larger trials are needed to confirm these findings. Thus, initiation of treatment later in gestation due to late entry into prenatal care could be considered. The majority of trials continue progesterone until either 36 completed weeks of gestation or delivery. Some providers choose to stop treatment at earlier gestational ages. Rebarber and coworkers[67] showed an increased incidence of recurrent preterm birth in women who stopped using 17-OHP-C before 32 weeks of gestation compared to women who continued until 36/6 weeks of gestation. It is unclear if stopping use at 33 to 35 weeks would confer equal risk.

Dose of Progesterone

The optimal dose of progesterone is unclear. Trials have varied widely in their dose amount and schedule of both vaginal progesterone and intramuscular 17-OHP-C. When opting for intramuscular progestin, the most widely studied dose is 250 mg weekly intramuscular 17-OHP-C. If opting for vaginal progesterone, a dose of either 100 to 200 mg micronized progesterone capsules vaginally nightly (compounded) or 90 mg Crinone 8% gel nightly would be reasonable.

Frequency of Use of Progesterone

A 2005 survey[68] of practicing maternal-fetal medicine specialists (n = 1264, 45% response rate) demonstrated that 67% used progesterone to prevent spontaneous preterm birth, with 38% of these using progesterone for other indications as well. Petrini and colleagues[69] reported that if were used on all eligible women, nearly 10,000 spontaneous preterm births could be prevented. This would amount to an overall reduction in the rate of preterm birth in the United States of approximately 2%.

Safety of Progesterone

Side effects
Side effects are fairly common with these drugs, including injection site reactions and urticaria. However, in only a few cases are they severe enough to lead to drug discontinuation. In the study of Rouse and colleagues,[39] more than 65% of women using 17-OHP-C experienced side effects, with most common being injection site reaction (61.6%) and urticaria (3.1%), but importantly leading to study drug discontinuation in only 0.6% patients. The most common complaint among users of vaginal progesterone is vaginal discharge, occurring in approximately 8% to 9% of patients, with approximately 4% attributable to the gel.[34]

Risk of congenital malformations

There is a large body of literature on the use of progestins in the first trimester for assisted reproduction. No teratogenic effects have been found.[70-72]

Risk of midtrimester loss

Many authors have raised concerns for the risk of midtrimester loss in women exposed to progesterone. In the original paper by Meis and colleagues,[32] the rate of spontaneous abortion was 5/306 women treated with 17-OHP-C compared to 0/153 placebo exposed patients (NS). The mean gestational age at study entry was 18.4 weeks. Although these data were not statistically significant, the trend for more stillbirth in the 17-OHP-C group (RR 1.5, 95% CI 0.3–7.4) raised concerns. Rouse and colleagues[39] also showed a nonsignificant trend toward an increase in fetal death rate in a group of twins whose mothers received 17-OHP-C (RR 1.4, 95% CI 0.6–3.2). In 2009, Norman and coworkers[38] also showed a trend toward increased fetal death in 17-OHP-C users (RR 1.5, 95% CI 0.5–4.4), with Combs and coworkers[41] having similar results in triplets. Conversely, Caritis and colleagues found a lower fetal death rate in a trial on triplets (RR 0.3, 95% CI 0.02–2.4).[40] In a Cochrane review,[73] there was not a statistically significant association with fetal death in any groups studied.

Risk for gestational diabetes

Few data exist on the risk for gestational diabetes mellitus (GDM) associated with progesterone. Progesterone is thought to contribute to the insulin resistance of pregnancy mainly through impaired beta-cell sensitivity to insulin and reduction in glucose transporter 4 expression.[74] In 2007, Rebarber and colleagues[75] raised the question in a retrospective cohort study of almost 600 women receiving 17-OHP-C and found a relative risk for the development of GDM of 2.9 (2.1,4.1). Again in 2009, Waters and colleagues[76] showed women taking 17-OHP-C to be at increased risk for GDM compared to those who did not take 17-OHP-C(RR 3.3, 95% CI 1.3–8.1). These studies both suggested a link. However, in 2009 Gyamfi and colleagues[77] published a secondary analysis of two RCTs of 17-OHP-C in both singleton and twin pregnancies and found no difference in the rates of GDM between women who were versus were not exposed to 17-OHP-C (adjusted OR 1.04, 95% CI 0.62–1.73). Thus, 17-OHP-C is not associated with the development of GDM. There are no trials on the rate of GDM in women exposed to vaginal progesterone.

Neonatal Outcomes

Many trials have included neonatal outcomes as part of their results. In a recent Cochrane review,[73] the only outcome shown to be significant was birth weight of less than 2500 g, with an RR of 0.64 [95% CI 0.49, 0.83]. In this meta-analysis, there was no difference for the outcomes of respiratory distress syndrome, intraventricular hemorrhage, retinopathy of prematurity, patent ductus arteriosus, fetal death, or neonatal death. Future trials will need to gather this information to elucidate an effect in these rare conditions with a larger sample size. There is very little long-term follow-up on these infants. Two-year follow-up data[78] from 278 children exposed to 17-OHP-C in utero show no difference in development. Longer term follow-up data are needed.

UNANSWERED QUESTIONS

Several unanswered questions exist surrounding the use of progestins for the prevention of preterm birth. Namely, the optimal route of administration, formulation, dose, and schedule have not been determined. In addition, long- term neonatal data

Table 2
Select ongoing trials for the use of progesterone for the prevention of preterm labor

Author	Title	Subjects	Intervention
Bruinse	17 alpha-Hydroxyprogesterone in multiple pregnancies to prevent handicapped infants (the AMPHIA Study)	Women with multiple pregnancy	Weekly IM 17-OHP-C vs placebo
Creasy	The effect of vaginal progesterone administration in the prevention of preterm birth in women with a short cervix. NCT00615550	Women with a singleton gestation and short cervical length (10–20 mm)	Daily vaginal progesterone vs placebo
Crowther	Progesterone for the prevention of neonatal respiratory distress syndrome (the PROGRESS Study). ISRCTN20269066	Women with a history of prior spontaneous preterm birth	Daily vaginal progesterone vs placebo
Grobman	RCT of progesterone to prevent preterm birth in nulliparous women with a short cervix. NCT00439374	Nulliparous women with a short cervix identified on transvaginal ultrasound	Weekly IM 17-OHP-C vs placebo
Martinez	Vaginal progesterone to prevent preterm delivery in women with preterm labor. NCT00536003	Women with signs of preterm labor and evidence of cervical change or positive fetal fibronectin testing.	Daily vaginal progesterone vs placebo
Maurel	17OHP for reduction of neonatal morbidity due to preterm birth in twin and triplet pregnancies. NCT00163020	Women with a twin or triplet pregnancy	Weekly IM 17-OHP-C vs placebo
Nassar	Prevention of preterm delivery in twin pregnancies by 17 alpha hydroxyprogesterone caproate. NCT00141908	Women with a twin pregnancy	Weekly IM 17-OHP-C vs placebo
Norman	Double blind randomised placebo controlled trial of progesterone for the prevention of preterm birth in twins. ISRCTN35782581	Women with a twin pregnancy	Daily vaginal progesterone vs placebo
Perlitz	Prevention of recurrent preterm delivery by a natural progesterone agent. NCT00329316	Women with preterm labor in prior pregnancy	Daily vaginal progesterone gel vs placebo
Rode	Does progesterone prevent very preterm delivery in twin pregnancies? NCT00329914	Women with a twin pregnancy	Daily vaginal progesterone vs placebo

Rozenberg	Efficacy of 17 alpha hydroxyl-progesterone caproate for the prevention of preterm delivery. NCT00331695	Women with either presentation in threatened preterm labor, history of prior preterm birth or multiple pregnancy (twins)	Weekly IM 17-OHP-C vs placebo
Serra	Natural progesterone and preterm birth in twins. NCT00480402	Women with a twin pregnancy	Natural progesterone vs placebo
Starkey	Comparing intramuscular versus vaginal progesterone for prevention of preterm birth. NCT00579553	Women with singleton pregnancies and history of prior spontaneous preterm birth	Weekly IM 17OHP (250 mg) vs daily vaginal progesterone (100mg)
Swaby	Pilot randomized controlled trial of vaginal progesterone to prevent preterm birth in multiple pregnancy	Women with a multiple pregnancy	Daily vaginal progesterone vs placebo
Wood	Vaginal progesterone versus placebo in multiple pregnancy. NCT0343265	Women with a multiple pregnancy	Daily vaginal progesterone gel vs placebo
Wood	Randomized controlled trial (RCT) of vaginal progesterone in women with threatened preterm labor (PIM). NCT01286246	Women 23–32/6 with arrested preterm labor or preterm ctx and +FFN	Daily vaginal progesterone vs placebo
Raed	Progesterone and second trimester bleeding NCT01269450	Women with second trimester bleeding	Daily vaginal progesterone vs placebo
Langen	Progesterone for maintenance tocolysis: a randomized placebo controlled trial. NCT00946088		Progesterone 400 mg per vagina qhs vs polyethylene glycol 400 distearate and hydrogenated vegetable oil
Palacio	Vaginal progesterone as a maintenance treatment in women with previous preterm labor: randomized, double blinded, placebo-controlled trial. NCT00646802		1 pessary, 200 mg, once daily since gestation age 36 weeks and 6 days
Reyes	Use of 17α hydroxyprogesterone caproate for the prevention of preterm labor in patients with a previous episode of threatened preterm labor during current pregnancy: double blind, randomized, controlled trial. NCT01317225		Weekly IM 17-OHP-C vs placebo

are needed. Lastly, more data are needed regarding maternal risks of progestin use, namely the risk of pregnancy loss. There are numerous ongoing trials on the use of progesterone for preterm delivery (**Table 2**). These will hopefully provide clarity on exactly who may benefit most from progesterone therapy, the optimal route, duration and dose of therapy, and if there ever should be a role for progesterone formulations in multiple gestation. In addition, the majority of women who have preterm delivery have no prior history of preterm birth. Whether there is a subset of these women who could be identified prospectively to benefit from progesterone is unknown.

SUMMARY OF RECOMMENDATIONS

Women with a history of prior spontaneous preterm birth, defined as delivery between 20/0 and 36/6 weeks of gestation due to either spontaneous preterm labor or PPROM, should be offered progesterone therapy.[53] Progesterone supplementation in women with a short cervix can be considered. There are no data to support the use of progesterone therapy in women with multiple gestation, women with PPROM, women with preterm labor, or women with a positive fetal fibronectin test.

The optimal dose, formulation, frequency, and timing of initiation for progestin therapy have not been determined. Based on prior trials, a dose of 250 mg of 17-OHP-C given weekly starting between 16/0 and 20/6 weeks of gestation and continued until 34 to 36 weeks gestation would be reasonable. Alternatively, the use of 100 to 200 mg intravaginal progesterone nightly or 90 mg intravaginal progesterone gel nightly could be considered.

There do not appear to be any significant maternal or fetal risks associated with progestin therapy. However, long-term neonatal follow-up data are still needed.

REFERENCES

1. Mathews TJ, MacDorman MF. Infant mortality statistics from the 2005 period linked birth/infant death data set. Natl Vital Stat Rep 2008;57(2):1–32.
2. Martin JA, Hamilton BE, Sutton PD, et al. Births: final data for 2007. Natl Vital Stat Rep 2010;58(24):1–85.
3. Hamilton BE, Martin JA, Ventura SJ. Births: Preliminary data for 2009. National Vital Statistics Report 2010;59(3):1–29.
4. J. Koppe, Ilsen A. Long-term outcome. London: Parthenon Publishing; 1998.
5. Centers for Disease Control and Prevention, National Center for Health Statistics. Final natality data. Hyattsville (MD): National Center for Health Statistics; 2008.
6. Morrison JC. Preterm birth: a puzzle worth solving. Obstet Gynecol 1990;76(Suppl I): 5S–12S.
7. Swamy GK, Ostbye T, Skjaerven R. Association of preterm birth with long-term survival, reproduction, and next-generation preterm birth. JAMA 2008;299(12): 1429–36.
8. Beck S, Wojdyla D, Say L, et al. The worldwide incidence of preterm birth: a systematic review of maternal mortality and morbidity. Bull World Health Organ 2010;88(1):31–8.
9. Joseph KS, Kramer MS, Marcoux S, et al. Determinants of preterm birth rates in Canada from 1981 through 1983 and from 1992 through 1994. N Engl J Med 1998;339(20):1434–9.
10. Dodd JM, Crowther CA, McPhee AJ, et al. Progesterone after previous preterm birth for prevention of neonatal respiratory distress syndrome (PROGRESS): a randomised controlled trial. BMC Pregnancy Childbirth 2009;9:6.
11. Moutquin JM. Classification and heterogeneity of preterm birth. BJOG 2003; 110(Suppl 20):30–3.

12. Sfakianaki AK, Norwitz ER. Mechanisms of progesterone action in inhibiting prematurity. J Matern Fetal Neonatal Med 2006;19(12):763–72.
13. Hegele-Hartung C, Chwalisz K, Beier HM, et al. Ripening of the uterine cervix of the guinea-pig after treatment with the progesterone antagonist onapristone (ZK 98.299): an electron microscopic study. Hum Reprod 1989;4(4):369–77.
14. Ruddock NK, Shi SQ, Jain S, et al. Progesterone, but not 17-alpha-hydroxyprogesterone caproate, inhibits human myometrial contractions. Am J Obstet Gynecol 2008;199(4):e391–7.
15. Csapo A. Progesterone block. Am J Anat 1956;98(2):273–91.
16. Allport VC, Pieber D, Slater DM, et al. Human labour is associated with nuclear factor-kappaB activity which mediates cyclo-oxygenase-2 expression and is involved with the 'functional progesterone withdrawal'. Mol Hum Reprod 2001;7(6):581–6.
17. Hardy DB, Janowski BA, Corey DR, et al. Progesterone receptor plays a major antiinflammatory role in human myometrial cells by antagonism of nuclear factor-kappaB activation of cyclooxygenase 2 expression. Mol Endocrinol 2006;20(11): 2724–33.
18. Condon JC, Jeyasuria P, Faust JM, et al. A decline in the levels of progesterone receptor coactivators in the pregnant uterus at term may antagonize progesterone receptor function and contribute to the initiation of parturition. Proc Natl Acad Sci USA 2003;100(16):9518–23.
19. Marx SG, Wentz MJ, Mackay LB, et al. Effects of progesterone on iNOS, COX-2, and collagen expression in the cervix. J Histochem Cytochem 2006;54(6):623–39.
20. Xu H, Gonzalez JM, Ofori E, et al. Preventing cervical ripening: the primary mechanism by which progestational agents prevent preterm birth? Am J Obstet Gynecol 2008; 198(3):e311–8.
21. Rajabi MR, Dodge GR, Solomon S, et al. Immunochemical and immunohistochemical evidence of estrogen-mediated collagenolysis as a mechanism of cervical dilatation in the guinea pig at parturition. Endocrinology 1991;128(1):314,1–8.
22. Ito A, Imada K, Sato T, et al. Suppression of interleukin 8 production by progesterone in rabbit uterine cervix. Biochem J 1994;301(Pt 1):183–6.
23. Foglia LM, Ippolito DL, Stallings JD, et al. Intramuscular 17alpha-hydroxyprogesterone caproate administration attenuates immunoresponsiveness of maternal peripheral blood mononuclear cells. Am J Obstet Gynecol 2010;203(6):561,e1–5.
24. Murtha AP, Feng L, Yonish B, et al. Progesterone protects fetal chorion and maternal decidua cells from calcium-induced death. Am J Obstet Gynecol 2007;196(3): 257.e1–5.
25. Cakmak H, Schatz F, Huang ST, et al. Progestin suppresses thrombin- and interleukin-1beta-induced interleukin-11 production in term decidual cells: implications for preterm delivery. J Clin Endocrinol Metab 2005;90(9):5279–86.
26. McLean M, Bisits A, Davies J, et al. A placental clock controlling the length of human pregnancy. Nat Med 1995;1(5):460–3.
27. Challis JR, Sloboda DM, Alfaidy N, et al. Prostaglandins and mechanisms of preterm birth. Reproduction 2002;124(1):1–17.
28. Jeschke U, Mylonas I, Richter DU, et al. Regulation of progesterone production in human term trophoblasts in vitro by CRH, ACTH and cortisol (prednisolone). Arch Gynecol Obstet 2005;272(1):7–12.
29. Karalis K, Goodwin G, Majzoub JA. Cortisol blockade of progesterone: a possible molecular mechanism involved in the initiation of human labor. Nat Med 1996;2(5): 556–60.
30. Levine L. Habitual abortion: a controlled study of progestational therapy. West J Surg Obstet Gynecol 1964;72:30–6.

31. Johnson JW, Austin KL, Jones GS, et al. Efficacy of 17alpha-hydroxyprogesterone caproate in the prevention of premature labor. N Engl J Med 1975;293(14):675–80.

32. Meis PJ, Klebanoff M, Thom E, et al. Prevention of recurrent preterm delivery by 17 alpha-hydroxyprogesterone caproate. N Engl J Med 2003;348(24):2379–85.

33. da Fonseca EB, Bittar RE, Carvalho MH, et al. Prophylactic administration of progesterone by vaginal suppository to reduce the incidence of spontaneous preterm birth in women at increased risk: a randomized placebo-controlled double-blind study. Am J Obstet Gynecol 2003;188(2):419–24.

34. O'Brien JM, Adair CD, Lewis DF, et al. Progesterone vaginal gel for the reduction of recurrent preterm birth: primary results from a randomized, double-blind, placebo-controlled trial. Ultrasound Obstet Gynecol 2007;30(5):687–96.

35. Briery CM, Veillon EW, Klauser CK, et al. Women with preterm premature rupture of the membranes do not benefit from weekly progesterone. Am J Obstet Gynecol 2011;204(1):54.e1–5.

36. Briery CM, Veillon EW, Klauser CK, et al. Progesterone does not prevent preterm births in women with twins. South Med J 2009;102(9):900–4.

37. Hartikainen-Sorri AL, Kauppila A, Tuimala R. Inefficacy of 17 alpha-hydroxyprogesterone caproate in the prevention of prematurity in twin pregnancy. Obstet Gynecol 1980;56(6):692–5.

38. Norman JE, Mackenzie F, Owen P, et al. Progesterone for the prevention of preterm birth in twin pregnancy (STOPPIT): a randomised, double-blind, placebo-controlled study and meta-analysis. Lancet 2009;373(9680):2034–40.

39. Rouse DJ, Caritis SN, Peaceman AM, et al. A trial of 17 alpha-hydroxyprogesterone caproate to prevent prematurity in twins. N Engl J Med 2007;357(5):454–61.

40. Caritis SN, Rouse DJ, Peaceman AM, et al. Prevention of preterm birth in triplets using 17 alpha-hydroxyprogesterone caproate: a randomized controlled trial. Obstet Gynecol 2009;113(2 Pt 1):285–92.

41. Combs CA, Garite T, Maurel K, et al. Failure of 17-hydroxyprogesterone to reduce neonatal morbidity or prolong triplet pregnancy: a double-blind, randomized clinical trial. Am J Obstet Gynecol 2010;203(3):248.e1–9.

42. Iams JD, Goldenberg RL, Meis PJ, et al. The length of the cervix and the risk of spontaneous premature delivery. National Institute of Child Health and Human Development Maternal Fetal Medicine Unit Network. N Engl J Med 1996;334(9):567–72.

43. Mercer BM, Goldenberg RL, Moawad AH, et al. The preterm prediction study: effect of gestational age and cause of preterm birth on subsequent obstetric outcome. National Institute of Child Health and Human Development Maternal-Fetal Medicine Units Network. Am J Obstet Gynecol 1999;181(5 Pt 1):1216–21.

44. DeFranco EA, O'Brien JM, Adair CD, et al. Vaginal progesterone is associated with a decrease in risk for early preterm birth and improved neonatal outcome in women with a short cervix: a secondary analysis from a randomized, double-blind, placebo-controlled trial. Ultrasound Obstet Gynecol 2007;30(5):697–705.

45. O'Brien JM, Defranco EA, Adair CD, et al. Effect of progesterone on cervical shortening in women at risk for preterm birth: secondary analysis from a multinational, randomized, double-blind, placebo-controlled trial. Ultrasound Obstet Gynecol 2009;34(6):653–9.

46. Fonseca EB, Celik E, Parra M, et al. Progesterone and the risk of preterm birth among women with a short cervix. N Engl J Med 2007;357(5):462–9.

47. Hassan SS, Romero R, Vidyadhari D, et al. Vaginal progesterone reduces the rate of preterm birth in women with a sonographic short cervix: a multicenter, randomized, double-blind, placebo-controlled trial. Ultrasound Obstet Gynecol 2011;38(1):18–31.

48. Owen J, Hankins G, Iams JD, et al. Multicenter randomized trial of cerclage for preterm birth prevention in high-risk women with shortened midtrimester cervical length. Am J Obstet Gynecol 2009;201(4):375.e1–8.
49. Keeler SM, Kiefer D, Rochon M, et al. A randomized trial of cerclage vs. 17 alpha-hydroxyprogesterone caproate for treatment of short cervix. J Perinat Med 2009; 37(5):473–9.
50. Berghella V, Figueroa D, Szychowski JM, et al. 17-Alpha-hydroxyprogesterone caproate for the prevention of preterm birth in women with prior preterm birth and a short cervical length. Am J Obstet Gynecol 2010;202(4):351.e1–6.
51. Durnwald CP, Momirova V, Rouse DJ, et al. Second trimester cervical length and risk of preterm birth in women with twin gestations treated with 17-alpha hydroxyprogesterone caproate. J Matern Fetal Neonatal Med 2010;23(12):1360–4.
52. Facchinetti F, Paganelli S, Comitini G, et al. Cervical length changes during preterm cervical ripening: effects of 17-alpha-hydroxyprogesterone caproate. Am J Obstet Gynecol 2007;196(5):453.e1–4 [discussion: 421].
53. ACOG Committee Opinion no. 419 October 2008 (replaces no. 291, November 2003). Use of progesterone to reduce preterm birth. Obstet Gynecol 2008;112(4): 963–5.
54. Gonzalez-Quintero VH, de la Torre L, Rhea DJ, et al. Impact of prior gestational age at preterm delivery on effectiveness of 17-alpha-hydroxyprogesterone caproate in practice. Am J Obstet Gynecol 2010;203(3):257,e1–5.
55. Rai P, Rajaram S, Goel N, et al. Oral micronized progesterone for prevention of preterm birth. Int J Gynaecol Obstet 2009;104(1):40–3.
56. Glover MM, McKenna DS, Downing CM, et al. A randomized trial of micronized progesterone for the prevention of recurrent preterm birth. Am J Perinatol 2011;28(5): 377–81.
57. Majhi P, Bagga R, Kalra J, et al. Intravaginal use of natural micronised progesterone to prevent pre-term birth: a randomised trial in India. J Obstet Gynaecol 2009;29(6): 493–8.
58. Bulletti C, de Ziegler D, Flamigni C, et al. Targeted drug delivery in gynaecology: the first uterine pass effect. Hum Reprod 1997;12(5):1073–9.
59. Cicinelli E, de Ziegler D, Bulletti C, et al. Direct transport of progesterone from vagina to uterus. Obstet Gynecol 2000;95(3):403–6.
60. De Ziegler D, Bulletti C, De Monstier B, et al. The first uterine pass effect. Ann NY Acad Sci 1997;828:291–9.
61. Cicinelli E, Borraccino V, Petruzzi D, et al. Pharmacokinetics and endometrial effects of the vaginal administration of micronized progesterone in an oil-based solution to postmenopausal women. Fertil Steril 1996;65(4):860–2.
62. Mahaguna V, McDermott JM, Zhang F, et al. Investigation of product quality between extemporaneously compounded progesterone vaginal suppositories and an approved progesterone vaginal gel. Drug Dev Ind Pharm 2004;30(10):1069–78.
63. Toner JP. Vaginal delivery of progesterone in donor oocyte therapy. Hum Reprod 2000;15(Suppl 1):166–71.
64. Silver RM, Cunningham FG. Deus ex Makena? Obstet Gynecol 2011;117(6):1263–5.
65. Gonzalez-Quintero VH, Istwan NB, Rhea DJ, et al. Gestational age at initiation of 17-hydroxyprogesterone caproate (17P) and recurrent preterm delivery. J Matern Fetal Neonatal Med 2007;20(3):249–52.
66. How HY, Barton JR, Istwan NB, et al. Prophylaxis with 17 alpha-hydroxyprogesterone caproate for prevention of recurrent preterm delivery: does gestational age at initiation of treatment matter? Am J Obstet Gynecol 2007;197(3):260,e1–4.

67. Rebarber A, Ferrara LA, Hanley ML, et al. Increased recurrence of preterm delivery with early cessation of 17-alpha-hydroxyprogesterone caproate. Am J Obstet Gynecol 2007;196(3):224,e1–4.

68. Ness A, Dias T, Damus K, et al. Impact of the recent randomized trials on the use of progesterone to prevent preterm birth: a 2005 follow-up survey. Am J Obstet Gynecol 2006;195(4):1174–9.

69. Petrini JR, Callaghan WM, Klebanoff M, et al. Estimated effect of 17 alpha-hydroxyprogesterone caproate on preterm birth in the United States. Obstet Gynecol 2005; 105(2):267–72.

70. Katz Z, Lancet M, Skornik J, et al. Teratogenicity of progestogens given during the first trimester of pregnancy. Obstet Gynecol 1985;65(6):775–80.

71. Resseguie LJ, Hick JF, Bruen JA, et al. Congenital malformations among offspring exposed in utero to progestins, Olmsted County, Minnesota, 1936–1974. Fertil Steril 1985;43(4):514–9.

72. Yovich JL, Turner SR, Draper R. Medroxyprogesterone acetate therapy in early pregnancy has no apparent fetal effects. Teratology 1988;38(2):135–44.

73. Dodd JM, Flenady VJ, Cincotta R, et al. Progesterone for the prevention of preterm birth: a systematic review. Obstet Gynecol 2008;112(1):127–34.

74. Branisteanu DD, Mathieu C. Progesterone in gestational diabetes mellitus: guilty or not guilty? Trends Endocrinol Metab 2003;14(2):54–6.

75. Rebarber A, Istwan NB, Russo-Stieglitz K, et al. Increased incidence of gestational diabetes in women receiving prophylactic 17alpha-hydroxyprogesterone caproate for prevention of recurrent preterm delivery. Diabetes Care 2007;30(9):2277–80.

76. Waters TP, Schultz BA, Mercer BM, et al. Effect of 17alpha-hydroxyprogesterone caproate on glucose intolerance in pregnancy. Obstet Gynecol 2009;114(1):45–9.

77. Gyamfi C, Horton AL, Momirova V, et al. The effect of 17-alpha hydroxyprogesterone caproate on the risk of gestational diabetes in singleton or twin pregnancies. Am J Obstet Gynecol 2009;201(4):392,e1–5.

78. Northen AT, Norman GS, Anderson K, et al. Follow-up of children exposed in utero to 17 alpha-hydroxyprogesterone caproate compared with placebo. Obstet Gynecol 2007;110(4):865–72.

Periodontal Disease and Preterm Birth

Amanda L. Horton, MD[a],*, Kim A. Boggess, MD[b]

KEYWORDS

- Infection • Inflammation • Periodontal disease
- Preterm birth

Preterm birth, defined as delivery at fewer than 37 weeks' gestation, is the most common cause of infant morbidity and mortality among nonanomalous infants in the United States. Preterm birth is responsible for 75% of neonatal mortality and 50% of long-term disability in children.[1,2] Approximately 20% of infant deaths are due to preterm birth, and survivors experience significant and life-long morbidity. Despite advances in basic, clinical, and translational research, as well as medical interventions to reduce preterm birth, the preterm birth rate has remained unchanged over the years.

Spontaneous preterm birth, which accounts for approximately 35% to 40% of all preterm births[3,4] results from a complex process of multiple etiologies. Important risk factors for spontaneous preterm birth are listed in **Box 1**.[4]

Maternal genitourinary and reproductive tract infections have been implicated as a risk factor in 15% to 25% of spontaneous preterm births.[5,6] Births that occur at less than 32 weeks gestation are more often complicated by infection than those at 32 weeks or greater,[6] and there is a higher rate of maternal inflammation and subclinical chorioamnionitis among births before 34 weeks.[7] Numerous investigators have shown an increased risk for preterm birth among women with bacterial vaginosis.[8–11] Research in the past decade has focused on associations between clinical infection, inflammation, and preterm birth. The risk of preterm birth with selected genitourinary tract infections is shown in **Table 1**.[12]

These findings have elucidated possible mechanisms in which infection and the subsequent inflammatory cascade can lead to preterm birth.[13] The associations between maternal genital and reproductive tract infection and preterm birth suggest that prevention or treatment of these infections would reduce preterm birth risk. However, trials treating maternal genital and reproductive tract infections to prevent

The authors have nothing to disclose.

[a] Northshore University Health System, Department of Maternal Fetal Medicine, Pritzker School of Medicine, University of Chicago, 2650 Ridge Avenue, Evanston, IL 60201-1718, USA

[b] Department of Maternal Fetal Medicine, University of North Carolina, CB 7570, Chapel Hill, NC 27599, USA

* Corresponding author.

E-mail address: amandamarder@gmail.com

Box 1
Risk factors for spontaneous preterm birth

Maternal age <18 or >40 years

African-American race

Previous preterm delivery

Smoking

Body mass index < 20 kg/m²

Low socioeconomic status

Multiple gestation

Maternal infection

---

preterm birth have been disappointing. For example, identification and treatment of bacterial vaginosis has inconsistently reduced preterm birth risk.[14–17]

Maternal infections distant from the reproductive tract have also been associated with preterm birth. Periodontal disease is a gram-negative, anaerobic of the mouth that occurs in 40% of pregnant women.[7] Infection and subsequent inflammation of the gingival and local support attachments of the teeth can result in tissue, bone, and ultimately, tooth loss. This destructive process involves both direct tissue damage from plaque bacterial products and indirect damage through bacterial stimulation of local and systemic inflammatory and immune responses.

More than a decade ago, Offenbacher and colleagues[18] reported a potential association between maternal periodontal infection and delivery of a preterm low birth weight infant. In a case-control study of 124 pregnant women, women who delivered at less than 37 weeks' gestation or an infant weighing less than 2500 g had significantly worse periodontal infection than control women.

Subsequently, 2 prospective cohort studies,[19,20] found that moderate-to-severe maternal periodontal infection identified early in pregnancy is associated with an increased risk of spontaneous preterm birth, independent of traditional risk factors. In the first study, Jeffcoat and co-workers[19] prospectively evaluated more than 1300 pregnant women.[19] Complete medical, behavioral, and periodontal data were collected between 21 and 24 weeks of gestation. Generalized periodontal infection was defined as 90 or more tooth sites with periodontal ligament attachment loss of 3 mm or more. The risk for preterm birth was increased among women with generalized periodontal infection; this risk was inversely related to gestational age. This relationship persisted after adjusting for maternal age, race, tobacco use, and parity, with the adjusted odds ratio (OR) for preterm birth before 37 weeks among women with

---

Table 1
Risk of preterm birth with selected genitourinary tract infection

Infection	Odds Ratio (95% Confidence Interval)
Bacterial vaginosis < 16 weeks	7.6 (1.8–31.7)
Neisseria gonorrhea	5.3 (1.6–17.9)
Asymptomatic bactiuria	2.1 (1.5–3.0)

generalized periodontal disease being 4.5 (95% confidence interval [CI], 2.2–9.2). The adjusted OR increased to 5.3 (95% CI, 2.1–13.6) for preterm birth at less than 35 weeks and to 7.1 (95% CI, 1.7–27.4) for preterm birth at fewer than 32 weeks of gestation.[19]

In the second study, Offenbacher and associates[20] prospectively examined obstetric outcomes of more than 1000 women who underwent both an antepartum and a postpartum periodontal examination. Moderate-to-severe periodontal infection was defined as 15 or more tooth sites with greater than 4 mm gingival pocket probing depths. The presence of worsening of periodontal infection, defined as clinical disease progression, was determined by comparing site-specific probing measurements between the antepartum and postpartum examinations. Disease progression was deemed present if 4 or more tooth sites demonstrated 2 mm or more increasing gingival pocket probing depth at each site, with the postpartum probing depth being 4 mm or greater. Compared with women with periodontal health, the relative risk (RR) for spontaneous preterm birth before 37 weeks' gestation was significantly elevated for women with moderate-to-severe periodontal infection (adjusted RR, 2.0; 95% CI, 1.2–3.2), adjusting for maternal age, race, parity, previous preterm birth, tobacco use, markers of socioeconomic status, and presence of chorioamnionitis. Periodontal disease progression was found to be an independent risk factor for delivery at fewer than 32 weeks (adjusted RR, 2.4; 95% CI, 1.1–5.2).[20] The findings from these 2 studies are notable, given the relationship between maternal periodontal disease and early preterm birth (less than 32 weeks of gestation), the significant neonatal morbidity and mortality associated with very preterm birth, and the prevention and treatment options available for periodontal infection.

The mechanism of periodontal disease association with preterm birth is not clear, but likely involves maternal and fetal inflammatory and immune response to the infectious burden. Maternal periodontal disease is association with a maternal inflammatory response, particularly among African-American women.[21] Fetal exposure to oral pathogens occurs,[22] and increases risk for preterm birth. This risk is even higher if there is also a fetal inflammatory response.[23] The mechanism may also involve translocation of oral bacteria to the amniotic cavity, and subsequent placental, uterine, or fetal responses that initiate preterm birth.[24,25]

The association of maternal periodontal infection and preterm birth led to intervention trials to determine whether identification and treatment of maternal periodontal disease reduced preterm birth risk. Early randomized, controlled trials suggested that maternal periodontal treatments during pregnancy may reduce the risk of spontaneous preterm birth.[26–28] Lopez and colleagues[26] conducted a randomized trial of 400 women with periodontal disease and compared periodontal treatment during pregnancy with delayed postpartum treatment. Periodontal disease was defined as 4 or more teeth with 1 or more sites with a pocket probing depth of 4 mm or greater and clinical attachment loss of 3 mm or greater. There was an almost a 5-fold reduction in preterm birth among women treated during pregnancy (OR, 5.49; 95% CI, 1.65–18.22). Periodontal disease was found to be an independent risk factor for spontaneous preterm birth (adjusted OR, 4.70; 95% CI, 1.29–17.13).[26]

In a pilot trial of periodontal treatment in 67 pregnant women, Offenbacher and associates[28] found a trend toward reduced preterm birth among women treated during pregnancy compared with those who delayed therapy until postpartum (adjusted OR, 0.26; 95% CI, 0.08–0.85). This study demonstrated significant improvement in oral health measures as well as a reduction in oral pathogen burden among women treated during pregnancy. Women treated during pregnancy had regression of clinical markers of periodontal infection, with reduction in tooth attachment loss and less bleeding on dental probing.[28]

Although early data suggested that identification and treatment of maternal periodontal disease reduced preterm birth, several large, randomized trials have failed to confirm this finding.[29–32] Michalowicz and colleagues[29] published the results of the Obstetrics and Periodontal Therapy Study, a multicenter, randomized trial of 823 pregnant women periodontal disease and compared periodontal treatment during pregnancy with delayed postpartum treatment conducted in the United States. Periodontal disease was defined as 4 or more teeth with a probing depth of at least 4 mm and a clinical attachment loss of at least 2 mm, as well as bleeding on probing at 35% or more of tooth sites. Although periodontal treatment during pregnancy did improve oral health parameters, it did not influence the risk of preterm birth (hazard ratio, 0.93; 95% CI, 0.63–1.37). In a subgroup analysis of women with severe periodontal disease, risk of preterm delivery did not differ significantly between the treatment and delayed treatment groups. However, a trend toward reduction in preterm birth before 32 weeks' gestation (2% vs 4%) was noted.[29]

Newnham and associates[30] conducted a single-center, randomized trial of 1000 pregnant women with periodontal disease and compared periodontal treatment during pregnancy with delayed postpartum treatment. Periodontal disease was defined as a probing pocket depth of 4 mm or more at 12 or more probing sites in fully erupted teeth. The preterm birth rates were similar between groups (9.7% in antepartum treatment vs 9.3% in delayed treatment group; OR, 1.05; 95% CI, 0.07–1.58). Significant improvements were noted in oral health parameters in women who underwent periodontal treatment.[30]

In the largest intervention trail to date of 1806 pregnant women, Offenbacher and co-investigators[31] conducted the Maternal Oral Therapy to Reduce Obstetric Risk study, a multicenter, randomized trial comparing antepartum periodontal treatment of scaling and root planning with delayed periodontal care after delivery. Periodontal disease was defined as at least 3 periodontal sites with at least 3 mm of clinical attachment loss in women with a minimum of 20 teeth. Similar to the previous smaller randomized studies, antepartum treatment did not reduce the incidence of preterm birth (13.1% in antepartum treatment vs 11.5% delayed treatment; $P = .316$). Oral health parameters did improve in women who received antepartum treatment and there was no increase in perinatal complications.[31]

More recently, Macones and co-workers[32] reported the results of the Periodontal Infections and Prematurity Study, a randomized trial of treatment of localized periodontal disease to reduce incidence of preterm birth. Periodontal disease was defined as clinical attachment loss of 3 mm or more on 3 or more teeth. Moderate-to-severe periodontal disease was defined as attachment loss of 5 mm or more on 3 or more teeth. The authors randomized 756 women to either active antepartum periodontal treatment, which consisted of scaling and root planning, or control treatment, which consisted of tooth polishing. The spontaneous preterm birth rate did not differ between groups: 5.3% in treatment group versus 4.4% in the control group. Active antepartum treatment did not reduce the risk of preterm delivery before 35 weeks of gestation (RR, 1.19; 95% CI, 0.62–2.25). In contrast to previous treatment trials, a greater proportion of women who received active treatment had a medically indicated preterm birth before 35 weeks' gestation compared with controls (3.3% vs 1.1%; RR, 3.01; 95% CI, 0.95–4.24).

In a recent systematic review and meta-analysis, Polyzos and associates[33] assessed whether treatment of periodontal disease with scaling and root planning during pregnancy is associated with a reduced rate of preterm birth. Eleven randomized controlled trials, in which 5 were considered to be of high methodologic quality, were included. The pooled results of the high-quality studies did not support a reductive in the risk of preterm birth (OR, 1.15; 95% CI, 0.95–1.40).[33]

The explanation for why treatment of maternal periodontal disease does not reduce preterm birth is unclear. One possibility is that maternal periodontal disease is merely a marker for another mechanism that is stimulating preterm birth. Another possible reason is that there is no consensus on the definition of periodontal disease and heterogeneity exists among different study populations. Periodontal disease and response to treatment in South America may differ from that in the United States or Australia. Another possible factor is the timing and frequency of periodontal treatment. All current, published, randomized, clinical trials tested periodontal treatment during pregnancy. Because periodontal disease is associated with local and systemic inflammation, treating periodontal disease during pregnancy may be too late to reduce the inflammatory burden that is associated with adverse pregnancy outcomes.[34] Periodontal treatment during pregnancy has usually been administered over 1 or 2 visits. Additional periodontal maintenance may be needed with advancing gestation.

Despite the lack of reduction in preterm birth, it is important to consider that treatment of maternal periodontal disease during pregnancy is not associated with any adverse maternal or fetal outcomes. In addition, the majority of treatment trials demonstrate that maternal oral health improves with antepartum periodontal therapy,[29–31] a finding that is important for overall maternal health and well-being.

In light of the data on maternal oral disease and pregnancy outcomes, clinicians should review with patients that oral health maintenance is an important part of preventive care and should be encouraged and supported before, during, and after pregnancy. Oral health interventions during pregnancy should be performed as general health maintenance, rather than to improve specific pregnancy outcomes.

REFERENCES

1. Markestad T, Kaaresen PI, Rønnestad A, et al. Early death, morbidity, and need of treatment among extremely premature infants. Pediatrics 2005;115:1289–98.
2. Mathews TJ, MacDorman MF. Infant mortality statistics from the 2005 period linked birth/infant death set. Natl Vital Stat Rep 2008;57:1–32.
3. Ananth CV, Vintzileos AM. Epidemiology of preterm birth and its clinical subtypes. J Matern Fetal Neonatal Med 2006;19:773782.
4. Goldenberg RL, Culhane JF, Iams JD, et al. Epidemiology and causes of preterm birth. Lancet 2008;371:75–84.
5. Romero R, Mazor M. Infection and preterm labor. Clin Obstet Gynecol 1988;31:533–84.
6. Goldenberg RL, Iams JD, Mercer BM, et al. The preterm prediction study: the value of new vs standard risk factors in predicting early and all spontaneous preterm births. NICHD MFMU Network. Am J Public Health 1998;88:233–8.
7. Lieff S, Boggess KA, Murtha AP, et al. The oral conditions and pregnancy study: periodontal status of a cohort of pregnant women. J Periodontol 2004;75:116–26.
8. Gravett MG, Nelson HP, DeRouen T, et al. Independent associations of bacterial vaginosis and Chlamydia trachomatis infection with adverse pregnancy outcome. JAMA 1986;256:1899–903.
9. Kurki T, Sivonen A, Renkonen OV, et al. Bacterial vaginosis in early pregnancy and pregnancy outcome. Obstet Gynecol 1992;80:173–7.

10. Holst E, Goffeng AR, Andersch B. Bacterial vaginosis and vaginal microorganisms in idiopathic premature labor and association with pregnancy outcome. J Clin Microbiol 1994;32:176–86.
11. Hillier SL, Nugent RP, Eschenbach DA, et al. Association between bacterial vaginosis and preterm delivery of a low- birth-weight infant. The Vaginal Infections and Prematurity Study Group. N Engl J Med 1995;333:1737–42.
12. Klein LL, Gibbs RS. Use of microbial cultures and antibiotics in the prevention of infection-associated preterm birth. Am J Obstet Gynecol 2004;190:1493–502.
13. Parry S, Strauss JS 3rd. Premature rupture of the fetal membranes. N Engl J Med 1998;338:663–70.
14. McGregor JA, French JI, Parker R, et al. Prevention of premature birth by screening and treatment for common genital tract infections: results of a prospective controlled evaluation. Am J Obstet Gynecol 1995;173:157–67.
15. McDonald HM, O'Loughlin JA, Vigneswaran R, et al. Impact of metronidazole therapy on preterm birth in women with bacterial vaginosis flora (Gardnerella vaginalis): a randomised, placebo controlled trial. Br J Obstet Gynecol 1997;104:1391–7.
16. Carey JC, Klebanoff MA, Hauth C, et al. Metronidazole to prevent preterm delivery in pregnant women with asymptomatic bacterial vaginosis. National Institute of Child Health and Human Development Network of Maternal-Fetal Medicine Units. N Engl J Med 2000;342:534–40.
17. Leitich H, Brunbauer M, Bodner-Adler B, et al. Antibiotic treatment of bacterial vaginosis in pregnancy: a meta-analysis. Am J Obstet Gynecol 2003;188:752–8.
18. Offenbacher S, Katz V, Fertik G, et al. Periodontal infection as a possible risk factor for preterm low birth weight. J Periodontol 1996;67(10 Suppl):1103–13.
19. Jeffcoat MK, Geurs NC, Reddy MS, et al. Periodontal infection and preterm birth: results of a prospective study. J Am Dent Assoc 2001;132:875–80.
20. Offenbacher S, Boggess KA, Murtha AP, et al. Progressive periodontal disease and risk of very preterm delivery. Obstet Gynecol 2006;107:29–36.
21. Horton AL, Boggess KA, Moss KL, et al. Periodontal disease early in pregnancy is associated with maternal systemic inflammation among African American women. J Periodontol 2008;79:1127–32.
22. Madianos PN, Lieff S, Murtha AP, et al. Maternal periodontitis and prematurity. Part II: Maternal infection and fetal exposure. Ann Periodontol 2001;6:175–82.
23. Boggess KA, Moss K, Madianos P, et al. Fetal immune response to oral pathogens and risk of preterm birth. Am J Obstet Gynecol 2005;193:1121–6.
24. Mikamo H, Kawazoe K, Sato Y, et al. Intra-amniotic infection caused by capnocytophaga species. Infect Dis Obstet Gynecol 1996;4:301–2.
25. Bearfield C, Davenport ES, Sivapathasundaram V, et al. Possible association between amniotic fluid micro-organism infection and microflora in the mouth. BJOG 2002;109: 527–33.
26. Lopez NJ, Smith PC, Guiterrez J. Periodontal therapy may reduce the risk of preterm low birth weight in women with periodontal disease: a randomized controlled trial. J Periodontol 2002;73:911–24.
27. Jeffcoat MK, Hauth JC, Guers NC, et al. Periodontal disease and preterm birth: results of a pilot intervention study. J Periodontol 2003;74:1214–8.
28. Offenbacher S, Lin D, Strauss R, et al. Effects of periodontal therapy during pregnancy on periodontal status, biologic parameters, and pregnancy outcomes: a pilot study. J Periodontol 2006;77:2011–24.
29. Michalowicz BS, Hodges JS, DiAngelis AJ, et al. Treatment of periodontal disease and the risk of preterm birth. N Engl J Med 2006;355:1885–94.

30. Newnham JP, Newnham IA, Ball CM, et al. Treatment of periodontal disease during pregnancy: a randomized controlled trial. Obstet Gynecol 2009;114:1239–48.
31. Offenbacher S, Beck J, Jared HL, et al. Effects of periodontal therapy on rate of preterm birth: a randomized controlled trial. Obstet Gynecol 2009;114:551–9.
32. Macones GA, Parry A, Nelson DB, et al. Treatment of localized periodontal disease in pregnancy does not reduce the occurrence of preterm birth: results from the periodontal infections and prematurity study (PIPS). Am J Obstet Gynecol 2010;202: 147,e1–8.
33. Polyzos NP, Polyzos IP, Zavos A, et al. Obstetric outcomes after treatment of periodontal disease during pregnancy: systematic review and meta-analysis. BMJ 2010;341:c7017.
34. Goldenberg RL, Culhane JF. Preterm birth and periodontal disease. N Engl J Med 2006;355:1925–7.

Cervical Cerclage for the Prevention of Preterm Birth

John Owen, MD, MSPH*, Melissa Mancuso, MD

KEYWORDS

• Cervical insufficiency • Cerclage • Risk factors
• Sonographic cervical length

Preterm birth continues to among the most problematic obstetrical issues, with an annually increasing incidence, now approaching 13% in the United States.[1] Most are not indicated for maternal/fetal complications, and so comprise the spontaneous preterm birth syndrome.[2] This syndrome includes multiple inciting factors, interrelated pathways, and several anatomic and related functional components; the underlying pathophysiology remains elusive and difficult to study. One anatomic component of this syndrome is the cervix, and when pathologic cervical changes predate uterine contractions or chorioamnion rupture, this has been clinically recognized as cervical insufficiency.

Although prior evidence suggested that cervical competence functions on a continuum of reproductive performance,[3–6] most women with a clinical diagnosis of cervical insufficiency have normal cervical anatomy, albeit with varying (presumably congenital) size or length. Thus, a poor reproductive history with a dominant cervical etiology more likely results from a process of premature cervical ripening (in the absence of clinical labor) caused by 1 or more underlying factors including subclinical infection in the decidua or amniotic cavity, local inflammation from noninfectious sources, hormonal effects, or even genetic predisposition, as women with certain progesterone receptor polymorphisms experience an increased risk of preterm birth.[7,8] When the integrity of the cervix becomes compromised, then additional processes may be stimulated, culminating in the preterm birth syndrome. In these cases, the process of preterm parturition seems to begin with the cervix and may be either accelerated or tempered by numerous other factors, many of which are obscure. Because the underlying mechanisms and interactions with the anatomic components associated with preterm birth are generally unknown, the specific timing of events leading to preterm birth cannot be determined. Therefore, prevention and treatment strategies have been largely empirically based and often ineffective.

Division of Maternal Fetal Medicine, Department of Obstetrics and Gynecology, University of Alabama, Birmingham, 1700 6th Avenue South, Women & Infants Center, Room 10270, Birmingham, AL 35233, USA
* Corresponding author.
E-mail address: johnowen@uab.edu

Obstet Gynecol Clin N Am 39 (2012) 25–33
doi:10.1016/j.ogc.2011.12.001
0889-8545/12/$ – see front matter © 2012 Elsevier Inc. All rights reserved.

CERCLAGE FOR RISK FACTORS

Four well-designed, randomized trials of history indicated (formerly called prophylactic) cerclage in women with "risk factors" for cervical insufficiency have been completed.[9–12] All but the largest[12] failed to show any benefit. This trial, performed by the Royal College of Obstetrics and Gynecology between 1981 and 1988, enrolled 1292 women who lacked a typical clinical history of insufficiency but whose managing physicians wondered whether cerclage might be indicated based on any of 6 historical risk factors. Delivery before 33 weeks' gestation was significantly lower (relative risk [RR], 0.75; 95% confidence interval [CI], 0.57–0.98) in cerclage-treated women than in controls. Because most untreated women delivered near term regardless, this benefit amounted to averting 1 preterm birth less than 33 weeks for every 25 treated with cerclage. Moreover, women in the cerclage group were more often treated with tocolytic agents, spent more time in the hospital, and experienced more puerperal fevers. In subgroup analyses, there was a significant reduction in the frequency of delivery before 33 weeks gestation only in the cohort of women with at least 3 prior second-trimester losses or preterm births. The authors concluded that this subgroup with the poorest obstetric history should undergo further study; however, this investigation was never performed. Thus, the available clinical trial data do not suggest a benefit for cerclage for risk factors except when the risk factor is recurrent (ie, ≥3) preterm births or second-trimester losses. Note that this trial predated the now commonly used cervical assessment with vaginal ultrasonography.

CERVICAL ULTRASONOGRAPHY AND THE PREDICTION OF PRETERM BIRTH

The assessment of cervical length has been well standardized,[13] is reproducible,[14] and provides useful information regarding at least 1 element of the preterm birth syndrome. Cervical length is an objective linear measurement that lends itself well to screening and identifying those at greatest risk for preterm birth.[15] Shortened cervical length is among the most powerful biologic markers of preterm birth and is most predictive when used in selected populations of high-risk gravidas, especially women with prior spontaneous preterm birth.

In 1996, Iams and colleagues[4] reported the results of a prospective, blinded, observational study of nearly 2000 unselected women. A strong inverse relationship between cervical length and the likelihood of spontaneous preterm birth before 35 weeks was reported. The associated positive predictive value for preterm births was only 18%; however, this was attributed to the unselected, low-risk population. This report demonstrated that cervical length screening was inefficient in low-risk, unselected populations.

In a subsequent blinded, observational trial, women at high risk for spontaneous preterm birth because of a prior spontaneous preterm birth before 32 weeks' gestation were studied.[15] Women whose cervical lengths were shorter than 25 mm had a relative risk of spontaneous preterm birth before 35 weeks of 4.5 (95% CI, 2.7–7.6). In logistic regression, for every 5 mm increase in the shortest observed cervical length, the odds of spontaneous preterm birth before 35 weeks fell by 43%. In a secondary analysis of this data, the authors hypothesized that spontaneous preterm birth should preferentially occur earlier in gestation if associated with shortened cervical length. In support of this, they observed an inverse relationship between cervical length and gestational age at birth: A shortened cervical length was preferentially associated with mid-trimester birth as opposed to third-trimester preterm birth.[16] These analyses suggest that shortened mid-trimester cervical length in women with a history of prior early spontaneous preterm birth implies a clinically significant component of diminished cervical competence (or alternatively, very early onset of parturition), which might be amenable to therapeutic intervention.

ULTRASONOGRAPHY-INDICATED CERCLAGE

Numerous investigators have reported that cervical insufficiency can be diagnosed by mid-trimester ultrasonographic evaluation of the cervix. Various ultrasonographic findings have been described and have been utilized to select women for treatment, generally cerclage.

Several randomized trials of cerclage for shortened cervical length (ultrasonography indicated) have been published.[17–22] Althuisius and colleageus[17] in 2001 published a 2-tiered, randomized trial of high-risk patients who were thought to have cervical insufficiency based on obstetric history or symptoms.[17] Women in the first tier were randomly allocated to prophylactic cerclage or cervical ultrasound surveillance. Thirty-five women in the ultrasound arm were found to have a shortened cervical length of less than 25 mm. These 35 women in the second tier underwent a second randomization to either cerclage or no cerclage. Both groups were instructed to use modified home rest. Of those women, 19 were assigned to cerclage and did not experience preterm birth before 34 weeks' gestation versus a 44% rate in the 16 women assigned to modified home rest without cerclage ($P = .002$). Importantly, no woman who maintained a cervical length of at least 25 mm experienced birth before 34 weeks. The outcomes were similar in those women who randomly underwent history-indicated (prophylactic) cerclage versus those women who were randomly assigned to undergo ultrasonography-indicated cerclage.

Rust and colleagues in 2001[18] completed a trial of 138 women who had various risk factors for preterm birth and who were randomly assigned to receive cerclage or not after their cervical length shortened to less than 25 mm or they developed funneling of more than 25%. The rate of preterm birth at fewer than 34 weeks' gestation in the cerclage group was 35% versus 36% in the no cerclage group ($P = .8$). In a large trial[19] of 47,123 unselected women, 470 were identified as having a shortened cervix of 15 mm or less. Of these, 253 participated in a randomized trial of Shirodkar cerclage (n = 127) versus no cerclage (n = 126). The primary outcome was the rate of delivery before 33 weeks' gestation. Here, there was no difference between groups with regard to the rate of preterm birth (22 vs 36%; $P = .44$). In another trial,[20] women with various risk factors for preterm birth, including prior preterm birth, dilation, and curettages, cone biopsy, and diethylstilbestrol exposure, underwent transvaginal ultrasound surveillance every 2 weeks from 14 to 23 weeks' gestation. Sixty-one experienced cervical length shortening of less than 25 mm or funneling greater than 25% and were randomized to McDonald cerclage versus no cerclage. Birth before 35 weeks' gestation occurred in 45% of the cerclage group and 47% of the control group ($P = .91$).

A patient-level meta-analysis[21] of these previously described 4 trials was performed by Berghella and colleagues in 2005 asking whether certain subgroups of women with mid-trimester cervical shortening might benefit from cerclage, defined as a relative risk reduction of preterm birth before 35 weeks' gestation. A marginal benefit was observed in singleton gestations, and the benefit was enhanced in those with a prior history of preterm birth (RR, 0.61; 95% CI, 0.4–0.9). These findings suggested that patients who experienced a prior spontaneous preterm birth attributed to other components of the spontaneous preterm birth syndrome might benefit from ultrasound-indicated cerclage for shortened cervical length.

To answer this specific question, a large, multicenter, randomized trial in high-risk women, defined as 1 or more prior early spontaneous preterm births at fewer than 34 weeks' gestation but who lacked a clinical history of cervical insufficiency, was recently completed.[22] A total of 1014 women underwent transvaginal ultrasonographic screening between 16 and 22 6/7 weeks' gestation. If the cervical length was at least 30 mm; scan frequency was every 2 weeks and increased to weekly when the cervical length was 25 to 29 mm. Those women whose cervical length shortened to less than 25 mm were randomly assigned to undergo McDonald cerclage or no cerclage. The primary outcome was the rate of preterm birth before 35 weeks' gestation.

Three hundred eighteen women (30%) developed cervical length shortening, and 302 consented to randomization. The rate of preterm birth in the no cerclage group was 42% versus 32% in the cerclage group (OR, 0.67; 95% CI, 0.42–1.07; $P = .09$). Survival analysis also demonstrated an improvement in overall pregnancy prolongation in the cerclage group ($P = .053$). In planned secondary analyses, birth before 37 weeks ($P = .01$), previable birth (at <24 weeks; $P = .03$), and perinatal mortality ($P = .046$) were less common in the cerclage group. As might be anticipated, there was a significant ($P = .03$) interaction between cervical length at randomization (<15 vs 15–24 mm) and assigned treatment, demonstrating a beneficial effect of cerclage in the shorter cervical length stratum, which was observed for both preterm birth (at <35 weeks; OR, 0.23; 95% CI, 0.08–0.66) and longer time to delivery in survival analysis ($P = .024$). The investigators concluded that, in women with a prior spontaneous preterm birth at less than 34 weeks' gestation and shortened cervical length to less than 25 mm between 16 and 22 6/7 weeks' gestation, cerclage did not show a benefit in preventing premature birth before 35 weeks, but did improve previable birth and perinatal mortality rates. The effect of cerclage for preventing preterm birth and prolonging gestation was most significant when the cervical length was less than 15 mm.

A more recent, patient-level meta-analysis published in 2011 by Berghella and colleagues[23] sought to estimate whether cerclage prevented preterm birth and perinatal mortality and morbidity in selected high-risk women, women with a prior spontaneous preterm birth, a singleton gestation, and a shortened cervical length. This meta-analysis included the same 4 trials as that discussed previously, but also included the multicenter, randomized trial of cerclage for preterm birth prevention.[22] Cerclage was found to significantly reduce preterm birth before 37, 32, 28, and 24 weeks of gestation. Although a composite outcome of either perinatal mortality or morbidity was also significantly reduced in the cerclage group (16%) versus the no cerclage group (25%; RR, 0.64; 95% CI, 0.45–0.91), preventing specific neonatal morbidities, alone or as a neonatal composite morbidity, has yet to be demonstrated.[23,24] Thus, the chief benefit of ultrasound-indicated cerclage for shortened cervical length in women with prior spontaneous preterm birth seems to be from preventing periviable births.[24]

CERVICAL ASSESSMENT BY ULTRASONOGRAPHY: BEYOND LENGTH

Other lower uterine segment and cervical characteristics in addition to cervical length can be assessed by mid-trimester ultrasonography. One of these characteristics is the presence of a cervical funnel. It has been shown that the presence of a funnel is a significant risk factor for adverse perinatal outcome and that it is best measured as a categorical variable (present or absent).[25] Other investigators have suggested that the finding of a funnel at the internal os is a poor independent predictor of preterm birth once the effect of short cervix is considered.[15] The shape of the funnel (U or V), percent funneling, and the depth and width of the funnel have all been described as methods of assessing cervical funneling. In high-risk women, the progression to a U-shaped funnel has been associated with an increased risk of preterm delivery.[25]

In a recent secondary analysis of the multicenter cerclage trial,[22] the effect of cervical funneling was evaluated.[26] Of the 301 women who comprised the study population,147 (49%) had a funnel present at their qualifying sonogram: 99 were V shaped and 48 were U shaped. In simple linear regression analysis, gestational age at delivery was found to differ significantly among the funnel groups ($P<.0001$). In particular, the presence of a U-shaped funnel differed from both V shaped ($P = .0003$) and no funnel ($P<.0001$). Rates of preterm birth before 24 weeks ($P = .004$), before 28 weeks ($P = .0004$), before 35 weeks ($P = .001$), and before 37 weeks ($P = .006$) differed among the funnel groups. Specifically, the presence of a U-shaped funnel (versus either V or none) was associated with preterm birth before 24 weeks ($P = .002$), before 28 weeks ($P = .0002$), before 35 weeks ($P = .0004$), and before 37 weeks ($P = .002$) gestation. There was no difference between no funnel and a V-shaped funnel for any preterm birth gestational age outcome. Time to delivery also differed significantly between funnel groups ($P = .0004$), where women with U-funnels demonstrated a significantly shorter time to birth than women with either a V-shaped funnel or no funnel ($P<.0001$). In the covariate-adjusted models, women with a U-shaped funnel continued to demonstrate significantly earlier gestational age at delivery ($P = .022$); women with a U-shaped funnel demonstrated earlier gestational age at delivery than women with either V-shaped ($P = .0123$) or no funnel ($P = .0077$). Women with a U-shaped funnel also demonstrated higher rates of preterm birth before 24, 28, 35, and 37 weeks.

THE BEST CERVICAL LENGTH CUTOFF FOR INTERVENTION

Debated among clinicians is the best cervical length for offering an ultrasound-indicated cerclage, because the continuum of preterm birth risk changes markedly at cervical lengths of less than 25 mm; the actual identification of this "optimal" cervical length cutoff for interventions remains problematic.[27] Both 15 and 25 mm have been utilized as action point cervical length cutoffs in randomized trials of cerclage. Another secondary analysis of the multicenter cerclage trial[22] was performed with the goal of defining an optimal cervical length for ultrasound-indicated cerclage in women with prior spontaneous preterm birth and short cervix (<25 mm).[27] The authors concluded that cerclage efficacy for preventing preterm birth varies both by the degree of cervical length shortening and the preterm birth gestational age threshold of interest. Nevertheless, for preventing preterm birth at thresholds of before 32 and before 35 weeks, cerclage efficacy improves steadily as cervical length shortens. At a previable preterm birth threshold of less than 24 weeks, cerclage remains effective down to a cervical length of 15 mm, below which it seems to lose some efficacy. Ultimately, the authors were unable to identify a single "best" or "optimal" cervical length for recommending ultrasound-indicated cerclage, but all cervical lengths between 15 and 24.9 mm seem to be appropriate for clinical use.

ADJUNCT THERAPY

Adjunct therapies to cerclage have been sought because ultrasound-indicated cerclage is not completely efficacious in women with a shortened cervical length. Some of these adjunct therapies include progesterone, indomethacin and antibiotics.[28,29]

Recently, the National Institute of Child Health and Human Development Maternal-Fetal Medicine Units Network reported the results of a double-blind trial of 17α-hydroxyprogesterone caproate for the prevention of spontaneous preterm birth in women with a prior spontaneous preterm birth.[30] Compared with placebo, weekly intramuscular injections reduced the rate of preterm birth by approximately one third. Current guidelines suggest the use of 17α-hydroxyprogesterone caproate in women with a prior spontaneous preterm birth,[31] and because essentially all women with a clinical history of cervical insufficiency have experienced this outcome, it should be considered as adjunct therapy.

Whether 17α-hydroxyprogesterone caproate is useful in women with shortened cervical length and a prior preterm birth has currently been studied. Berghella and associates[32] published a planned secondary analysis of the National Institute of Child Health and Human Development–sponsored randomized trial evaluating cerclage from high-risk women with shortened cervical length. Their objective was to estimate the effect of 17-OH-progesterone caproate (17P) for the prevention of preterm birth in women with prior spontaneous preterm birth, short cervical length, with and without ultrasound-indicated cerclage. They concluded that 17P had no additional benefit for prevention of preterm birth in women who have prior spontaneous preterm birth and receive ultrasound-indicated cerclage for cervical length of less than 25 mm. In women who do not undergo cerclage, 17P did reduce previable birth and perinatal mortality rates.

The clinical scenario of ultrasonographic short cervix in women with no prior history of preterm birth is one not infrequently encountered. The question of the best treatment modality in this setting has scarce data. To help answer this question, Hassan and colleagues[33] performed a multicenter, randomized trial that enrolled asymptomatic women with a singleton pregnancy and shortened cervical length (10–20 mm) on ultrasonography to determine the efficacy and safety of using daily micronized vaginal progesterone (90 mg) gel to reduce preterm birth.[33] They found that the administration of vaginal progesterone gel to women with an ultrasonographic short cervix in the mid trimester was associated with a 45% reduction in the rate of preterm birth. Additionally, there was decreased neonatal morbidity and mortality and no differences in the incidence of treatment-related adverse events between the groups.[33]

Tocolytic therapy, specifically indomethacin, has also been studied as an adjunct to cerclage therapy. Vinsintine and co-workers[28] published a retrospective cohort study of asymptomatic women with an ultrasound-indicated cerclage placed because of a short cervical length (<25 mm). Indomethacin therapy consisted of 50 mg administered orally or rectally followed by 25 mg given orally every 6 hours for approximately 48 hours. Of 101 participants, 51 women received indomethacin at the time of cerclage placement and 50 women did not. There was no difference in the rate of preterm birth at fewer than 35 weeks in those women who received indomethacin at the time of cerclage placement versus those who did not. The rates of spontaneous preterm birth were also similar at fewer than 32 weeks' gestation (RR, 1.1; 95% CI, 0.6–1.9). Logistic regression analysis showed that indomethacin administration at the time of ultrasound-indicated cerclage was not an independent predictor of spontaneous preterm birth. The authors concluded that, although there was no difference in the rates of preterm birth, randomized trials were indicated.

Other adjunct therapies include antibiotic use at the time of ultrasound-indicated cerclage. Antibiotics are commonly used, but there is no data to support their efficacy. Prophylactic antibiotics at the time of cerclage would be used to theoretically reduce a surgical site infection, because acute cervicitis and chorioamnionitis are contraindications to cerclage placement. Shiffman[29] in 2001 reported a study of 10 women with history of failed cerclage in prior pregnancy with short cervical length and funneling in the current pregnancy that underwent ultrasound-indicated cerclage.

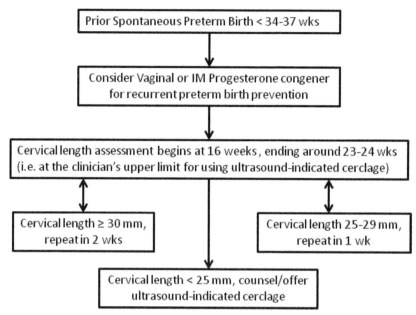

Fig. 1. Flowchart for cervical length assessment and ultrasonography-guided cerclage.

These women were continuously treated with low-dose antibiotics. The outcome was number of weeks of pregnancy gained in the index pregnancy minus the weeks of the prior pregnancy. All 10 achieved fetal viability. Pregnancy was prolonged by a mean of 13.4 ± 4.2 weeks beyond the previous pregnancy ($P<.001$). The authors concluded that continuous low-dose antibiotics prolong pregnancy in patients with recurrent second-trimester pregnancy losses and prior failed cerclage. The findings of this small study notwithstanding, larger confirmatory clinical trials are needed to define the role of prophylactic antibiotics in these high-risk pregnancies.

SUMMARY

Contemporary evidence supports the concept that cervical insufficiency is anything but a well-defined and distinct clinical entity. Instead, it is only 1 component of the larger and more complex preterm birth syndrome. Premature cervical ripening, as evidenced by shortening and effacement beginning at the internal os, provides strong evidence that parturition has begun and is the result of multiple interrelated pathways and inciting factors. Ultrasonographic screening of the cervix and treatment with cerclage for cervical shortening in the mid-trimester is reserved for women with prior spontaneous preterm birth (**Fig. 1**). Although cerclage benefit increases as the cervix shortens to less than 25 mm, it is appropriate to offer cerclage to women with shortened cervical length of less than 25 mm, and particularly those with a coexistent U-shaped funnel.

REFERENCES

1. Martin JA, Hamilton BE, Sutton PD, et al. Centers for Disease Control and Prevention National Center for Health Statistics National Vital Statistics System. Births: Final data for 2005. Nat Vital Stat Rep 2007;56(6);1–103.

2. Romero R, Espinoza J, Kusanovic JP, et al. The preterm parturition syndrome. Br J Obstet Gynaecol 2006;113(Suppl 3):17–42.
3. Iams JD, Johnson FF, Sonek J, et al. Cervical competence as a continuum: a study of ultrasonographic cervical length and obstetric performance. Am J Obstet Gynecol 1995;172:1097–106.
4. Iams JD, Goldenberg RL, Meis PJ, et al; for the National Institute of Child Health and Human Development Maternal Fetal Medicine Unit Network. The length of the cervix and the risk of spontaneous premature delivery. N Engl J Med 1996;334:567–72.
5. Buckingham JC, Buethe RA, Danforth DN. Collagen-muscle ratio in clinically normal and clinically incompetent cervixes. Am J Obstet Gynecol 1965;91:232–7.
6. Ayers JWR, DeGrood RM, Compton AA, et al. Sonographic evaluation of cervical length in pregnancy: diagnosis and management of preterm cervical effacement in patients at risk for premature delivery. Obstet Gynecol 1988;71:939–44.
7. Manuck TA, Lai Y, Meis PJ, et al. Progesterone receptor polymorphisms and clinical response to 17-alpha-hydroxyprogesterone caproate. Am J Obstet Gynecol 2011;205:135.e1–9.
8. Mancuso MS, Lobashevsky E, Biggio J. Response to 17-α-hydroxyprogesterone is affected by progesterone receptor polymorphisms. Am J Obstet Gynecol 2011;204:S24–5 (#43).
9. Dor J, Shalev J, Mashiach S, et al. Elective cervical suture of twin pregnancies diagnosed ultrasonically in the first trimester following induced ovulation. Gynecol Obstet Invest 1982;13:55–60.
10. Lazar P, Gueguen S, Dreyfus J, et al. Multicentered controlled trial of cervical cerclage in women at moderate risk of preterm delivery. Br J Obstet Gynaecol 1984;91:731–5.
11. Rush RW, Isaacs S, McPherson K, et al. A randomized controlled trial of cervical cerclage in women at high risk for preterm delivery. Br J Obstet Gynaecol 1984;91:724–30.
12. Anonymous. Final report of the Medical Research Council/Royal College of Obstetrics and Gynecology multicentre randomized trial of cervical cerclage. Br J Obstet Gynaecol 1993;100:516–23.
13. Sonek J, Shellhaas C. Cervical sonography: a review. Ultrasound Obstet Gynecol 1998;11:71–8.
14. Burger M, Weber-Rossler T, Willmann M. Measurement of the pregnant cervix by transvaginal sonography: an interobserver study and new standards to improve the interobserver variability. Ultrasound Obstet Gynecol 1997;9:188–93.
15. Owen J, Yost N, Berghella V, et al; for the National Institute for Child Health and Human Development Maternal Fetal Medicine Unit Network. Mid-trimester endovaginal sonography in women at high risk for spontaneous preterm birth. JAMA 2001;286:1340–8.
16. Owen J, Yost N, Berghella V et al. Can shortened mid-trimester cervical length predict very early spontaneous preterm birth? Am J Obstet Gynecol 2004;191:298–303.
17. Althuisius SM, Dekker GA, Hummel P, et al. Final results of the cervical incompetence prevention randomized cerclage trial (CIPRACT): therapeutic cerclage with bed rest versus bed rest alone. Am J Obstet Gynecol 2001;185:1106–12.
18. Rust OA, Atlas RO, Reed J, et al. Revisiting the short cervix detected by transvaginal ultrasound in the second trimester: why cerclage may not help. Am J Obstet Gynecol 2001;185:1098–105.
19. To MS, Alfirevic Z, Heath VCF, et al; on behalf of the Fetal Medicine Foundation Second Trimester Screening Group. Cervical cerclage for prevention of preterm delivery in women with short cervix: randomized controlled trial. Lancet 2004;363:1849–53.

20. Berghella V, Odibo AO, Tolosa JE. Cerclage for prevention of preterm birth in women with a short cervix found on transvaginal ultrasound: a randomized trial. Am J Obstet Gynecol 2004;191:1311–7.
21. Berghella V, Odibo AO, To MS, et al. Cerclage for short cervix on ultrasonography, meta-analysis of trials using individual patient-level data. Obstet Gynecol 2005;106: 181–9.
22. Owen J, Hankins G, Iams JD, et al. Multicenter randomized trial of cerclage for preterm birth prevention in high-risk women with shortened mid-trimester cervical length. Am J Obstet Gynecol 2009;201:375.e1–8.
23. Berghella V, Rafael TJ, Szychowski JM, et al. Cerclage for short cervix on ultrasonography in women with singleton gestations and previous preterm birth. A meta-analysis. Obstet Gynecol 2011;117:663–71.
24. Owen J, Szychowski J; for the Vaginal Ultrasound Trial Consortium. Neonatal morbidities in a multicenter randomized trial of ultrasound-indicated cerclage for shortened cervical length. Am J Obstet Gynecol 2011;204:S17–8.
25. Berghella V, Owen J, MacPherson C, et al; National Institute of Child Health and Human Development (NICHD) Maternal-Fetal Medicine Units Network (MFMU). Natural history of cervical funneling in women at high risk for spontaneous preterm birth. Obstet Gynecol 2007;109:863–9.
26. Mancuso MD, Szychowski JM, et al; Vaginal Ultrasound Trial Consortium. Cervical funneling: effect on gestational length and ultrasound-indicated cerclage in high-risk women. Am J Obstet Gynecol 2010;203:259,e1–5.
27. Owen J, Szychowski J; for the Vaginal Ultrasound Trial Consortium. Can the optimal cervical length for placing ultrasound-indicated cerclage be identified? Am J Obstet Gynecol 2011;204:S198–9.
28. Vinsintine J, Airoldi J, Berghella V. Indomethacin administration at the time of ultrasound-indicated cerclage: is there an association with a reduction in spontaneous preterm birth? Am J Obstet Gynecol 2008;198:643,e1–643.e3.
29. Shiffman RL. Continuous low-dose antibiotics and cerclage for recurrent second-trimester pregnancy loss. J Reprod Med 2000;45:323–6.
30. Meis PJ, Klebanoff M, Thom E, et al. Prevention of recurrent preterm birth by 17 alpha-hydroxyprogesterone caproate. NEJM 2003;348:2379–85.
31. ACOG Committee Opinion No 419: October 2008. Use of progesterone to reduce preterm birth.
32. Berghella V, Figueroa D, Szychowski JM, et al; Vaginal Ultrasound Trial Consortium. 17-Alpha-hydroxyprogesterone caproate for the prevention of preterm birth in women with prior preterm birth and a short cervical length. Am J Obstet Gynecol 2010;202: 351.e1–6.
33. Hassan SS, Romero R, Vidyadhari D, et al. Vaginal Progesterone reduces the rate of preterm birth in women with a sonographic short cervix: a multicenter, randomized, double-blind, placebo-controlled trial. Ultrasound Obstet Gynecol 2011;38:18–31.

Late Preterm Birth: Management Dilemmas

Cynthia Gyamfi-Bannerman, MD

KEYWORDS

- Late preterm birth • Prematurity • Respiratory morbidity
- Management

BACKGROUND AND EPIDEMIOLOGY

In 2005 the phrase "late preterm" was introduced by the National Institute of Child Health and Human Development (NICHD) to characterize infants born between 34 0/7 and 36 6/7 weeks of gestation as a high-risk group with increased morbidities when compared with term infants. This replaced the earlier phrase "near term," which implied these infants behaved similarly to term infants. Limiting this group to neonates born from 34 to 36 weeks also helped focus research on this cohort, allowing investigators to better characterize their outcomes. We now have ample data that show most morbidities related to prematurity are increased in the late preterm group when compared with infants born at term, most markedly where respiratory morbidities are concerned.[1–3] This heightened awareness of adverse outcomes raises the question of whether delivery in this period for a variety of indications can be avoided. The focus of this article is a description of the epidemiology and management of late preterm pregnancy.

Late preterm birth has contributed to the shift in the average gestational age at birth from 40 weeks to 39 weeks, and it has driven the increase in prematurity. In 1981, 6.3% of births occurred in the late preterm period.[4] This rate increased steadily to 9.1% in 2005–2006, where it peaked, representing a 30.1% increase from 1981.[5] The rise in late preterm birth was a result of several factors. In the early 1990s, there were data to show that most morbidities related to prematurity were significantly decreased by 34 weeks of gestation.[6,7] These data, along with the 1994 NIH Consensus Statement that discouraged the use of steroids beyond 34 weeks because of the low risk of respiratory distress syndrome (RDS) and lack of data to show benefit, inadvertently encouraged obstetricians to deliver patients beyond 34 weeks for a variety of indications without concern for neonatal outcomes.[8]

The preliminary data on births from 2009 suggest that late preterm birth has declined by 5% from 2006 to 8.7%.[9] These data, along with the unprecedented

The author has nothing to disclose.

Division of Maternal-Fetal Medicine, Columbia University Medical Center, 622 West 168th Street, New York, NY 10032, USA

E-mail address: cg2231@columbia.edu

Obstet Gynecol Clin N Am 39 (2012) 35–45
doi:10.1016/j.ogc.2011.12.005
0889-8545/12/$ – see front matter © 2012 Published by Elsevier Inc.

obgyn.theclinics.com

Table 1
RDS, TTN by gestational week

Gestational Age (weeks)	RDS % (n)	TTN % (n)
34	6.4 (41/636)	11.9 (76/636)
35	4.1 (39/945)	6.9 (65/945)
36	1.2 (20/1702)	3.6 (62/1702)
Term (≥37)	0.09 (53/58427)	0.42 (244/58427)

Data from Rubaltelli FF, Dani C, Reali MF, et al and Italian Group of Neonatal Pneumology. Acute neonatal respiratory distress in Italy: a one-year prospective study. Acta Paediatr 1998;87:1261–8.

2-year decrease in the rate of all prematurity, are promising. Whether the decline is related to new obstetric interventions or a lack of intervention is yet to be determined.

LATE PRETERM MORBIDITY
Respiratory Morbidity

Some of the earliest data are from Rubaltelli and colleagues, who conducted a study of more than 65,000 infants born over a 1-year period that showed that neonatal respiratory morbidity, as well as other morbidities, were inversely related to gestational age.[10] This trend persisted even for those born in the late preterm period (**Table 1**).

More recently, McIntire and Leveno reviewed late preterm respiratory morbidities over an 18- year period at Parkland Medical Center.[2] They identified 21,771 late preterm births, accounting for 9% of total births and 76% of preterm births. Specific respiratory morbidities, including ventilator use and transient tachypnea of the newborn (TTN), were higher in late preterm versus term infants (**Fig. 1**). Yoder and colleagues also quantified the frequency of respiratory disease in late preterm infants.[1] Respiratory morbidity from all causes was higher at 34 weeks (22%), 35 weeks (8.5%), and 36 weeks (3.9%) when compared to 39 and 40 weeks (0.7% and 0.8%, respectively, *P*<.001). It should be noted that the differences in respiratory morbidity rates between these two studies are due to institution-specific definitions of respiratory distress and TTN.

Finally, in 2010 the Safe Labor Consortium evaluated respiratory morbidity associated with late preterm delivery in a cohort of women who delivered in the late

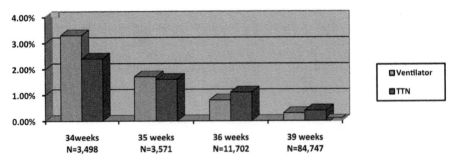

Fig. 1. Respiratory morbidity in late preterm pregnancy compared with term. (*Data from* McIntire DD, Leveno KJ. Neonatal mortality and morbidity rates in late preterm births compared with births at term. Obstet Gynecol 2008;111:35–41.)

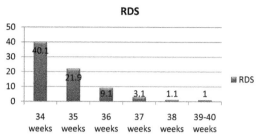

Fig. 2. Adjusted odds of RDS by gestational age at birth. (*Data from* Hibbard JU, Wilkins I, Sun L, et al. Respiratory morbidity in late preterm births. JAMA 2010;304:419–25.)

preterm period over 8 years.[3] They found an increase in the rate of RDS, TTN, pneumonia, respiratory failure, surfactant use, and ventilator use that also inversely correlated to the gestational age at delivery. Specifically, RDS was 40-fold higher at 34 weeks compared with 39 weeks (odds ratio [OR] 40.1; 95% confidence intervals [CI] 32.0, 50.3) (**Fig. 2**), while neonatal intensive care unit (NICU) admission was 11 times more common at 34 weeks (67.4%) compared to 39 weeks (6.1%).

Other Late Preterm Morbidities

An infant born very preterm is at an increased risk for a number of acute medical complications, including intraventricular hemorrhage (IVH), necrotizing enterocolitis (NEC), patent ductus arteriosus (PDA), and sepsis. Although these complications diminish as term approaches and organ systems mature, within the late preterm birth group several neonatal morbidities remain higher compared with term births. In addition to respiratory morbidity, these include sepsis, hyperbilirubinemia requiring phototherapy, and IVH (**Fig. 3**).

LATE PRETERM MORTALITY

Reddy and colleagues evaluated neonatal mortality rates among late preterm infants delivered without a recorded indication[11] (**Table 2**). They found neonatal mortality rates of 7.1, 4.8, and 2.8 respectively at 34 weeks, 35 weeks, and 36 weeks gestation. More concerning was that the increased neonatal morbidity persisted into the 37th week with a 1.7 per 1000 mortality rate at this gestational age. Tomashek and

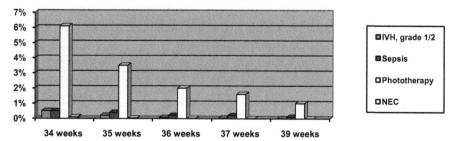

Fig. 3. Nonrespiratory morbidity among late preterm infants compared with infants born at 39 weeks. (*Data from* McIntire DD, Leveno KJ. Neonatal mortality and morbidity rates in late preterm births compared with births at term. Obstet Gynecol 2008;111:35–41.)

Table 2
Neonatal and infant mortality rates (2001): deaths per 1000 births

Gestational Age (weeks)	Neonatal Mortality Rate	RR (95% CI)	Infant Mortality Rate	RR (95% CI)
34	7.1	9.5 (8.4, 10.8)	11.8	5.4 (4.9, 5.9)
35	4.8	6.4 (5.6, 7.2)	8.6	3.9 (3.6, 4.3)
36	2.8	3.7 (3.3, 4.2)	5.7	2.6 (2.4, 2.8)
37	1.7	2.3 (2.1, 2.6)	4.1	1.9 (1.8, 2.0)
38	1.0	1.4 (1.3, 1.5)	2.7	1.2 (1.2, 1.3)
39	0.8	1.0 (reference)	2.2	1.0 (reference)
40	0.8	1.0 (0.9, 1.1)	2.1	0.9 (0.9, 1.0)

Data from Reddy UM, Ko CW, Raju TN, et al. Delivery indications at late-preterm gestations and infant mortality rates in the United States. Pediatrics 2009;124:234–40.

colleagues found similar rates in a cohort of late preterm infants born over a 7-year period.[4] There was an increase in early, late, and overall infant mortality of six times, two times, and three times that of term mortality rates, respectively.

LONG-TERM LATE PRETERM OUTCOME DATA

Long-term data on neurologic outcomes associated with late preterm delivery are limited, but the available information is also concerning. Moster and colleagues linked gestational age at delivery to the rate of medical disability in a group of adults born between 1967 and 1983 in Norway.[12] They found that infants delivered between 34 and 36 weeks of gestation were 2.7 times more likely to have cerebral palsy, 1.6 more times likely to have mental retardation, and 1.5 times more likely to have disorders of psychological development, behavior, and emotion compared with infants born at term. The findings of Morse and colleagues were similar to these. They evaluated a group of school-aged children in Florida who were born in the late preterm period and found that the children were more likely to have developmental delay and disability in pre-kindergarten, require a "special needs" education, and experience suspension in kindergarten (**Table 3**).[13] Although many late preterm deliveries are unavoidable, these data should caution again elective delivery in this gestational age window.

Table 3
Early school-age outcomes of LP infants in FL (n = 161,804)

Early School-Age Outcome	Healthy Late Preterm (%)	Term (%)	Adjusted RR
Developmental delay/disability	4.24	2.96	1.36 (1.29–1.43)
Disability in pre–kindergarten	7.40	6.60	1.10 (1.05–1.14)
Not ready to start school	5.09	4.40	1.04 (1.00–1.09)
"Special needs" education	13.30	11.88	1.10 (1.07–1.13)
Retention in kindergarten	7.96	6.17	1.11 (1.07–1.15)
Suspension in kindergarten	1.80	1.22	1.19 (1.10–1.29)

Data from Morse SB, Zheng H, Tang Y, et al. Early school-age outcomes of late preterm infants. Pediatrics 2009;123:e622–9.

MANAGEMENT OF LATE PRETERM PREGNANCY

Because of the known morbidity and mortality associated with late preterm birth, iatrogenic delivery in this period has become a major concern. Preterm birth has traditionally been characterized as either "spontaneous" (preterm labor or preterm premature rupture of the membranes [PPROM]) or "indicated." For the most part, spontaneous late preterm births are difficult to avoid, whereas the term "indicated" implies that the delivery was necessary for some maternal or fetal benefit. However, particularly in the late preterm population, some of the indicated deliveries can best be characterized as elective.[11,14,15] It follows that a decrease in the elective rate of late preterm deliveries can in turn decrease the rate of many late preterm complications.

It is difficult to characterize a late preterm delivery as indicated versus elective. There are many regional differences in practice that may result in a varied number of accepted indications. For example, Holland and coworkers reviewed 514 late preterm births at their institution over a 1-year period.[14] They found that fewer than10% of those deliveries were elective. Interestingly, included in their "indicated" category were deliveries for mild preeclampsia, intrauterine growth restriction (IUGR) with normal fetal testing, and prior stillbirth. The authors acknowledged that their classification of the appropriateness of delivery was based on limited scientific evidence and commented that within their own group, they debated the appropriateness of each indication. Another approach to assessing indications for delivery in this gestational age window is to classify the births as evidence based or non-evidence based. Gyamfi-Bannerman and colleagues used this approach and found that 56.7% of late preterm nonspontaneous deliveries were non-evidence based, concluding that more data were needed to justify many indications.[15] Recently, recommendations on appropriate late preterm deliveries were published from the 2011 workshop cosponsored by the Society for Maternal-Fetal Medicine and the National Institute of Child Health and Human Development entitled "Timing of Indicated Late Preterm and Early Term Births."[16] Diagnoses for which late preterm delivery was considered appropriate included suspected accreta, monochorionic/diamniotic twin gestation, fetal growth restriction with a comorbidity such as oligohydramnios, or abnormal Doppler studies. Interestingly, the suggested gestational age for delivery for a prior stillbirth was at 39 weeks of gestation, and not in the late preterm period as suggested by Holland and colleagues.[14] The authors from the workshop commented that most of their recommendations were based on grade B evidence (limited or inconsistent scientific evidence).[16]

Although curtailing the pathophysiology resulting in preterm labor or PPROM may not be possible, whether expeditious delivery is warranted, particularly after PPROM, has been newly debated. The question of whether a delay in delivery beyond 34 weeks is harmful for patients with PPROM was recently addressed by a review in the Cochrane database of the use of antibiotics with ruptured membranes. They showed that administration of antibiotics significantly decreased the rates of both neonatal infection (OR 0.67; 95% CI 0.52, 0.85) and chorioamnionitis (OR 0.66; 95% CI 0.46, 0.96) at up to 37 weeks of gestation.[17] Patients who were included in this review delivered at up to 37 weeks of gestation. Another Cochrane database review of expectantly managed PPROM to 37 weeks of gestation showed that there were no differences in the rates of neonatal sepsis (risk ratio [RR] 1.33; 95% CI 0.72, 2.47), perinatal mortality (RR 0.98; 95% CI 0.41, 2.36), intrauterine deaths (RR 0.26; 95% CI 0.04, 1.52), or neonatal deaths (RR 1.59; 95% CI 0.61, 4.16) when comparing early delivery with expectant management.[18] Interestingly, early delivery increased the incidence of cesarean delivery (RR 1.51; 95% CI 1.08, 2.10) and endometritis (RR

2.32; 95% CI 1.33, 4.07), likely secondary to a higher cesarean delivery rate in that group. However, there was no statistical difference in the rates of chorioamnionitis (RR 0.44; 95% CI 0.17, 1.14), suggesting safety with short-term delay. Ongoing prospective trials, including PPROMT and PPROMEXIL, will help to elucidate further whether prolonged expectant management to 37 weeks of gestation is appropriate for late preterm PPROM.[19,20]

OBSTETRIC COMPLICATIONS
Hypertensive Disorders of Pregnancy

There is some debate and regional variation regarding the appropriate gestational age for delivery of patients with some of the hypertensive disorders of pregnancy. Although most experts agree that patients with clinically stable severe preeclampsia should be delivered by 34 weeks or less of gestation, the appropriate gestational age for delivery of patients with mild preeclampsia and gestational hypertension are more nebulous. A recent clinical trial evaluating labor induction versus expectant management for mild preeclampsia and gestational hypertension at 36 weeks or greater found that maternal outcomes were improved with labor induction after 37 weeks.[21] The authors did not find this trend with delivery between 36 and 37 weeks, but they cited low numbers in that subgroup as a reason for further study at that gestational age. Habli and coworkers performed a secondary analysis of data from an NICHD clinical trial on calcium to prevent preeclampsia.[22] Specifically, they tried to assess whether the poorer neonatal outcomes related to gestational hypertension and preeclampsia were secondary to the disease process or iatrogenic delivery resulting from these diagnoses in a cohort of both hypertensive and normotensive women delivering at 35, 36, or 37 weeks of gestation. The authors found a higher rate of small for gestational age, NICU admission, and neonatal length of stay in the hypertensive compared with the normotensive group. These differences did not vary by the severity of hypertension; rather, they seemed to be related to labor induction. The authors concluded that the need for intervention at these earlier gestational ages should be carefully evaluated. Recently, Barton and colleagues reviewed outcomes specifically associated with gestational hypertension and late preterm delivery using a retrospective database.[23] They found that elective delivery from 34 to 36 weeks of gestation resulted in increased neonatal morbidity without maternal benefit. The cited literature suggests that patients with mild preeclampsia or gestational hypertension can be delivered at term ($\geq$37 weeks). The NICHD/Society for Maternal-Fetal Medicine (SMFM) workshop had a similar conclusion recommending delivery at 37 weeks for mild preeclampsia and 37 to 38 weeks for gestational hypertension.[16]

Oligohydramnios

Another common diagnosis that often leads to delivery in the late preterm period is oligohydramnios, defined commonly as either an amniotic fluid index (AFI) of less than 5 or an AFI that is less than the 5th percentile for gestational age. Much of the literature suggesting increased neonatal morbidity in the setting of oligohydramnios does not account for existing comorbidities that can influence the perinatal outcome.[24,25]

Zhang and colleagues found a population of women with isolated oligohydramnios and evaluated the correlation with this finding and perinatal morbidity.[26] Using data from the Routine Antenatal Diagnostic Imaging with UltraSound (RADIUS) trial in which women underwent routine ultrasound screening, they identified a population of 113 women with isolated oligohydramnios. There was no association with adverse perinatal outcomes in this group of women. The NICHD/SMFM workshop recommendation for timing of delivery with pregnancies complicated by isolated oligohydramnios is intervention between 36 and 37 weeks of gestation.

Placenta Accreta

Placenta accreta is a potentially life-threatening condition characterized by abnormal invasion of the placenta into the myometrium, usually at the level of a prior uterine scar. The decision as to when to deliver these patients is based on weighing the potential benefit of pregnancy continuation for the neonate in preventing iatrogenic prematurity against the risk of maternal labor and hemorrhage necessitating emergent delivery and thereby increasing the likelihood of complications. Designing a clinical trial to answer these questions is difficult at best, partly because of the relatively low incidence of this complication. Because of these limitations, Robinson and Grobman designed a decision analysis for optimal delivery timing. They found that a scheduled delivery at 34 weeks of gestation resulted in the highest quality-adjusted life years for both mother and neonate. Further, there was no additional benefit when fetal lung maturity testing was added to the model. The SMFM clinical opinion paper on placenta accreta states that planned late preterm delivery (34 0/7–36 6/7 weeks of gestation) is an acceptable management strategy because there are data showing increased rates of hemorrhage once delivery occurs beyond 36 weeks of gestation.[27]

Prior Classic Cesarean

Although the timing of an elective repeat cesarean after a prior low transverse cesarean is clear at 39 weeks of gestation, it is less clear when the prior scar was a classic uterine incision. The rate of uterine rupture in women with a prior classic scar is thought to be between 4% and 9%.[28] Chauhan and colleagues reviewed uterine rupture and dehiscence rates in a cohort of 157 women who had a prior classic cesarean.[29] All were planned for repeat cesarean. There was one uterine rupture in this series, and it was of a woman who presented with bleeding at 29 weeks of gestation. The rupture resulted in an intrauterine fetal demise (IUFD). Otherwise, there was a 9% dehiscence rate noted at the time of repeat cesarean, which did not alter maternal or neonatal outcomes compared with the women without dehiscence. Interestingly, almost 50% of these patients presented in preterm labor before an amniocentesis could be done to document fetal lung maturity. Although the mean duration of labor was 7.3 ± 5.6 hours, there were no uterine ruptures in that group. The authors concluded that uterine rupture and dehiscence could not be predicted accurately or prevented. Other data not specific to classic cesarean comes from a review of more than 40,000 deliveries in a hospital in Ireland.[30] Of the 1355 women with one or more prior cesarean deliveries attempting a trial of labor, 6 experienced uterine ruptures. There was one pre-labor rupture in a woman with a prior classic cesarean, but the authors did not provide information on how many patients had had a prior classic cesarean. There is very little other evidence to help guide timing of delivery in these patients. Expert opinion regarding timing of delivery in these cases remains delivery before the onset of labor. This is consistent with the recommendation from the NICHD/SMFM workshop for delivery at 36 to 37 weeks of gestation.

Twin Gestation

It is known that women with twin gestations deliver earlier than those with singletons, with the average gestational age of delivery thought to be in the late preterm period.[31] However, there are very few indications for elective delivery of dichorionic, diamniotic twins in this gestational age window outside of coexisting maternal or obstetric complications warranting delivery. The consensus of the NICHD/SMFM workshop participants regarding elective late preterm delivery for dichorionic twins was in the situation of an IUFD of a co-twin.

However, the appropriate gestational age for delivery of uncomplicated monochorionic, diamniotic (mono/di) twins is highly debated. The recommendations vary from 32 weeks to 37 weeks gestation.[32–35] Barigye and colleagues identified a group of 151 uncomplicated mono/di twin gestations and evaluated the risk of fetal demise.[32] They found that the risk of IUFD at 32 weeks of gestation or greater in these seemingly normal twins was 1 in 23. Further, 4.6% of pregnancies had an IUFD within 2 weeks of a normal scan. They suggested that a policy of elective preterm delivery at 32 weeks of gestation or greater would negate this risk. On the other end of the spectrum, Smith and colleagues reviewed 236 ongoing mono/di twin pregnancies and found that the likelihood of 2 live births in the "uncomplicated" group was 99.5% at 32 weeks or greater.[34] They recommended against elective preterm delivery of uncomplicated mono/di twins. Consensus and expert opinion suggest delivery for uncomplicated mono/di twins should occur in the late preterm period between 34 and 37 weeks of gestation.[16]

The Role of Amniocentesis

We now have ample data that show respiratory morbidity remains higher in infants delivered at late preterm gestations when compared to 39 weeks. Bates and colleagues performed a retrospective review of 459 neonates delivered after documented fetal lung maturity from 36 0/7 weeks to 38 6/7 weeks of gestation. The authors evaluated a composite of possible complications including neonatal death, RDS, TTN, bronchopulmonary dysplasia, persistent pulmonary hypertension, need for respiratory support (including ventilator support or any other mode of supplemental oxygenation), use of surfactant, metabolic complications including hypoglycemia, hyperbilirubinemia requiring treatment, generalized seizures, necrotizing enterocolitis, hypoxic ischemic encephalopathy periventricular leukomalacia, feeding difficulties, and suspected or proven sepsis. They found that the incidence of the composite outcome decreased with increasing gestational age (P for trend <.001): 9.2% (CI 5.9%, 14.1%) at 36 weeks, 3.2% (CI 1.5%, 6.8%) at 37 weeks, 5.2% (CI 2.0%, 12.6%) at 38 weeks, and 2.5% (CI 2.2%, 2.8%) at 39–40 weeks. Even beyond 36 weeks of gestation, although fetal lung maturity testing may reliably exclude RDS, it does not predict other important morbidities. Therefore, mature results may not predict adverse outcomes. The role of amniocentesis was discussed at the NICHD/SMFM workshop on timing of delivery.[16] The consensus was that if there was significant maternal or fetal risk that warranted delivery, amniocentesis would not further aid in guiding management. The converse was also thought to be true. If delivery could be delayed to await pulmonary maturity, then the indication is less urgent and prompt delivery is not likely indicated.

Potential Role of Corticosteroids

The landmark study by Liggins and Howie that first described the use of betamethasone to induce fetal pulmonary maturity included patients at risk for preterm delivery from 24 to 37 weeks of gestation.[36] When they analyzed their data by gestational age at delivery, there was a trend toward a decrease in the rate of RDS if the women were delivered between 32 and less than 37 weeks of gestation, but this number did not reach statistical significance (4.7% (2/43) vs 6.9% (2/29), NS [P-value not reported]). Because of the small numbers of affected infants in this cohort, they were likely underpowered to show a difference in this subgroup. Similarly, a Cochrane database review analyzing rates of RDS after antenatal corticosteroid administration found that if the initial dose was given at 35 to less than 37 weeks of gestation, there was a trend toward a benefit of this treatment (RR 0.61; 95% CI 0.11, 3.61), but the finding was also not statistically significant.[37] All of the patients included in that particular subgroup analysis were from the original Liggins and Howie study. Of note, there were only 6 cases of RDS in the cohort of 189 patients, 2 in the betamethasone group, and 4 in the control group. Again, this was likely underpowered to show benefit. However, if the first dose of steroids was given from 33 to more than 35 weeks of gestation (which includes a late preterm population), there was a significant decrease in the rate of RDS in the treatment group (RR 0.53; 95% CI 0.31, 0.91).

One recent study evaluated the ability of antenatal corticosteroids to reduce respiratory morbidity in a late preterm cohort.[38] Patients were randomized to betamethasone or placebo, and the primary outcome of either RDS or TTN was compared between groups. They found no difference in the rate of the primary outcome, but acknowledge that they were underpowered to evaluate RDS. There was also a lower rate of the primary outcome in the placebo group than anticipated, which likely relates to the numbers of infants who delivered at term. Currently, there is an ongoing randomized, clinical trial by the Maternal-Fetal Medicine Units Network to evaluate whether antenatal corticosteroids reduce respiratory morbidity in late preterm infants (Clinical Trials.gov Identifier: NCT01222247).

Future Research in Late Preterm Birth

There are many potential areas for research in the area of late prematurity. As noted previously, whether antenatal corticosteroids will help to reduce the respiratory morbidity associated with birth in this time period has yet to be determined. In lieu of the increased awareness of morbidity and mortality associated with late preterm birth, indications for delivery during this time period need to be systematically assessed for risks versus benefits of late preterm delivery. Further data on long-term outcomes including the potential for developmental delay and other neurologic sequelae are needed.

SUMMARY

In summary, late preterm birth results from spontaneous, indicated, and sometime elective indications. The burden of prematurity can be decreased if elective late preterm delivery is eliminated. While recent recommendations from the NICHD/SMFM workshop on timing of late preterm and early term birth have helped to guide management, the authors acknowledge that most of their guidelines are based on grade B or C evidence. Certain conditions absolutely warrant late preterm delivery; however, the clinician should weigh the risks of iatrogenic prematurity with the benefits of delivery for maternal or fetal indication when considering intervention for this cohort.

REFERENCES

1. Yoder BA, Gordon MC, Barth WH Jr. Late-preterm birth: does the changing obstetric paradigm alter the epidemiology of respiratory complications? Obstet Gynecol 2008; 111:814–22.
2. McIntire DD, Leveno KJ. Neonatal mortality and morbidity rates in late preterm births compared with births at term. Obstet Gynecol 2008;111:35–41.
3. Hibbard JU, Wilkins I, Sun L, et al. Respiratory morbidity in late preterm births. JAMA 2010;304:419–25.

4. Tomashek KM, Shapiro-Mendoza CK, Davidoff MJ, et al. Differences in mortality between late-preterm and term singleton infants in the United States, 1995–2002. J Pediatr 2007;151:450–6, 6 e1.
5. Late preterm births: US 1998–2008. Available at http://www.marchofdimes.com/peristats/level1.aspx?dv=ls&reg=99&top=3&stop=240&lev=1&slev=1&obj=1. Accessed August 18, 2011.
6. Copper RL, Goldenberg RL, Creasy RK, et al. A multicenter study of preterm birth weight and gestational age-specific neonatal mortality. Am J Obstet Gynecol 1993; 168:78–84.
7. Robertson PA, Sniderman SH, Laros RK Jr, et al. Neonatal morbidity according to gestational age and birth weight from five tertiary care centers in the United States, 1983 through 1986. Am J Obstet Gynecol 1992;166:1629–41 [discussion: 1641–5].
8. NIH Consensus Development Panel on Optimal Calcium Intake. NIH Consensus Conference. Optimal calcium intake. JAMA 1994;272:1942–8.
9. Hamilton BE, Martin JA, Ventura SJ. Births: preliminary data for 2009. Natl Vital Stat Rep 2010;59:1–19.
10. Rubaltelli FF, Dani C, Reali MF, et al and Italian Group of Neonatal Pneumology. Acute neonatal respiratory distress in Italy: a one-year prospective study. Acta Paediatr 1998;87:1261–8.
11. Reddy UM, Ko CW, Raju TN, et al. Delivery indications at late-preterm gestations and infant mortality rates in the United States. Pediatrics 2009;124:234–40.
12. Moster D, Lie RT, Markestad T. Long-term medical and social consequences of preterm birth. N Engl J Med 2008;359:262–73.
13. Morse SB ZH, Tang Y, Roth J. Early school-age outcomes of late preterm infants. Pediatrics 2009;123:e622–9.
14. Holland MG, Refuerzo JS, Ramin SM, et al. Late preterm birth: how often is it avoidable? Am J Obstet Gynecol 2009;201:404. e1–4.
15. Gyamfi-Bannerman C, Fuchs K, Young O, et al. Non-spontaneous late preterm birth: etiology and outcomes. Am J Obstet Gynecol 2011;205:456.e1–6.
16. Spong CY, Mercer BM, D'Alton M, et al. Timing of indicated late-preterm and early-term birth. Obstet Gynecol 2011;118:323–33.
17. Kenyon S, Boulvain M, Neilson JP. Antibiotics for preterm rupture of membranes. Cochrane Database Syst Rev 2010;8:CD001058.
18. Buchanan SL, Crowther CA, Levett KM, et al. Planned early birth versus expectant management for women with preterm prelabour rupture of membranes prior to 37 weeks' gestation for improving pregnancy outcome. Cochrane Database Syst Rev 2010;3:CD004735.
19. Morris JM, Roberts CL, Crowther CA, et al. Protocol for the immediate delivery versus expectant care of women with preterm prelabour rupture of the membranes close to term (PPROMT) Trial [ISRCTN44485060]. BMC Pregnancy Childbirth 2006;6:9.
20. van der Ham DP, Nijhuis JG, Mol BW, et al. Induction of labour versus expectant management in women with preterm prelabour rupture of membranes between 34 and 37 weeks (the PPROMEXIL-trial). BMC Pregnancy Childbirth 2007;7:11.
21. Koopmans CM, Bijlenga D, Groen H, et al. Induction of labour versus expectant monitoring for gestational hypertension or mild pre-eclampsia after 36 weeks' gestation (HYPITAT): a multicentre, open-label randomised controlled trial. Lancet 2009; 374:979–88.
22. Habli M, Levine RJ, Qian C, et al. Neonatal outcomes in pregnancies with preeclampsia or gestational hypertension and in normotensive pregnancies that delivered at 35, 36, or 37 weeks of gestation. Am J Obstet Gynecol 2007;197:406.e1–7.

23. Barton JR, Barton LA, Istwan NB, et al. Elective delivery at 34(/) to 36(/) weeks' gestation and its impact on neonatal outcomes in women with stable mild gestational hypertension. Am J Obstet Gynecol 2011;204:44.e1–5.

24. Casey BM, McIntire DD, Bloom SL, et al. Pregnancy outcomes after antepartum diagnosis of oligohydramnios at or beyond 34 weeks' gestation. Am J Obstet Gynecol 2000;182:909–12.

25. Hsieh TT, Hung TH, Chen KC, et al. Perinatal outcome of oligohydramnios without associated premature rupture of membranes and fetal anomalies. Gynecol Obstet Invest 1998;45:232–6.

26. Zhang J, Troendle J, Meikle S, et al. Isolated oligohydramnios is not associated with adverse perinatal outcomes. BJOG 2004;111:220–5.

27. Belfort MA. Placenta accreta. Am J Obstet Gynecol 2010;203:430–9.

28. Cunningham FG Levino K, Bloom SL, et al. Williams obstetrics. 23rd edition. New York: McGraw-Hill; 2010.

29. Chauhan SP, Magann EF, Wiggs CD, et al. Pregnancy after classic cesarean delivery. Obstet Gynecol 2002;100:946–50.

30. Meehan FP, Magani IM. True rupture of the caesarean section scar (a 15 year review, 1972–1987). Eur J Obstet Gynecol Reprod Biol 1989;30:129–35.

31. Malone FD, D'Alton ME. Multiple gestation: clinical characteristics and management. In: Greene MF, Creasy RK, Resnik R, et al, editors. Creasy and Resnik's maternal-fetal medicine: principles and practice. 6th edition. Philadelphia: Saunders Elsevier; 2009. p. 453–76.

32. Barigye O, Pasquini L, Galea P, et al. High risk of unexpected late fetal death in monochorionic twins despite intensive ultrasound surveillance: a cohort study. PLoS Med 2005;2:e172.

33. Hack KE, Derks JB, Elias SG, et al. Increased perinatal mortality and morbidity in monochorionic versus dichorionic twin pregnancies: clinical implications of a large Dutch cohort study. BJOG 2008;115:58–67.

34. Smith NA, Wilkins-Haug L, Santolaya-Forgas J, et al. Contemporary management of monochorionic diamniotic twins: outcomes and delivery recommendations revisited. Am J Obstet Gynecol 2010;203:133.e1–6.

35. Lee YM, Wylie BJ, Simpson LL, et al. Twin chorionicity and the risk of stillbirth. Obstet Gynecol 2008;111:301–8.

36. Liggins GC, Howie RN. A controlled trial of antepartum glucocorticoid treatment for prevention of the respiratory distress syndrome in premature infants. Pediatrics 1972;50:515–25.

37. Roberts D, Dalziel S. Antenatal corticosteroids for accelerating fetal lung maturation for women at risk of preterm birth. Cochrane Database Syst Rev 2006;3:CD004454.

38. Porto AM, Coutinho IC, Correia JB, et al. Effectiveness of antenatal corticosteroids in reducing respiratory disorders in late preterm infants: randomised clinical trial. BMJ 2011;342:d1696.

Antenatal Corticosteroids in the Management of Preterm Birth: Are We Back Where We Started?

Clarissa Bonanno, MD*, Ronald J. Wapner, MD

KEYWORDS

- Corticosteroids • Preterm birth • Prematurity
- Neonatal mortality • Respiratory distress

TRENDS IN PRETERM BIRTH

For nearly three decades, the preterm birth rate has been steadily increasing in the United States, rising by more than 30% during this time period.[1] However, after peaking at 12.8% of all births in 2006, the preterm birth rate has declined for three consecutive years, to 12.18% in 2009.[2] As preterm birth can result in serious long-term medical and developmental problems, with tremendous individual, family, and societal cost, this represents a most welcome trend. Meeting the *Healthy People 2020* goal of an 11.4% rate of preterm birth may now be possible.

The reasons for this recent downtrend in preterm birth are not entirely clear. The decrease has been demonstrated in both late preterm (34–36 completed weeks) deliveries and early preterm deliveries (<34 weeks).[2] Preterm births for patients delivered by cesarean, induced vaginal birth, and noninduced vaginal birth have all declined,[3] and the reduction in preterm birth is not explained by a change in the proportion of multiple births.[3] These data suggest that efforts by the American Congress of Obstetricians and Gynecologists (ACOG) and other advocacy groups such as the March of Dimes have helped to decrease iatrogenic late preterm birth. In addition, interventions such as 17α-hydroxyprogesterone caproate for prevention of recurrent preterm birth and vaginal progesterone for prevention of preterm birth in women with a short cervix may be effectively reducing the rate of spontaneous preterm birth.

Even with the recent decline, preterm birth remains a critical public health issue in this country. Primary prevention of preterm birth remains the ultimate goal. However,

The authors have nothing to disclose.

Division of Maternal Fetal Medicine, Department of Obstetrics and Gynecology, Columbia University College of Physicians and Surgeons, 161 West 168th Street, New York, NY 10032, USA
* Corresponding author.
E-mail address: cab90@columbia.edu

Obstet Gynecol Clin N Am 39 (2012) 47–63
doi:10.1016/j.ogc.2011.12.006
0889-8545/12/$ – see front matter © 2012 Elsevier Inc. All rights reserved.

until a better understanding of the mechanisms underlying preterm birth leads to its effective and universal prevention, efforts to minimize the impact of preterm birth on neonatal morbidity and mortality are paramount. Antenatal corticosteroid treatment for fetuses born preterm remains one of the most important antenatal interventions in obstetric practice.

HISTORICAL PERSPECTIVE

The story of antenatal corticosteroids—the discovery of this therapy for fetal maturation, the adoption into clinical practice, and the evolution of corticosteroid administration in obstetrics—highlights several fascinating and universal truths about science and medicine. The first is that scientific breakthroughs are often happened upon incidentally. In the 1960s, the obstetrician Graham Liggins was investigating factors involved in the initiation of labor in a sheep model. His goal was to solve the problem of preterm labor by determining what controls labor at term. While testing his hypothesis that steroid hormones might trigger labor, he found that preterm lambs exposed to corticosteroids in utero had structurally more mature lungs, were viable at an earlier gestational age, and had less severe respiratory distress at birth than expected.[4] The pediatrician Ross Howie helped Liggins appreciate the potential for this therapy to improve the lung function in premature infants. Liggins and Howie then designed and conducted a randomized controlled trial (RCT) on maternal administration of betamethasone. The results were published in a landmark article in 1972.[5] Not only did this therapy reduce the incidence of respiratory distress syndrome (RDS) in preterm infants from 15.6% to 10.0%, but further analysis showed a reduction in neonatal mortality from 11.6% to 6.0%.[6]

The second point that the story of corticosteroids illustrates is that clinicians can be slow to adopt new therapies into clinical practice. Over the next few decades, additional studies corroborated the findings of Liggins and Howie. However, concerns about the quality of the evidence and fears about potential side effects made obstetric providers hesitant to use this therapy routinely for women at risk for preterm birth.[7,8] In 1990, Crowley and colleagues published a meta-analysis of 12 RCTs of antenatal corticosteroids, demonstrating that this therapy significantly reduced RDS and other neonatal morbidities such as intraventricular hemorrhage (IVH) and necrotizing enterocolitis (NEC) as well as overall neonatal mortality.[9] In 1994 the National Institutes of Health (NIH) held a consensus conference to review the safety and efficacy of antenatal corticosteroids. Based on the recent meta-analysis and other available evidence, the panel recommended that antenatal corticosteroids be administered to all women at risk for preterm birth between 24 and 34 weeks' gestation.[10] This recommendation and the endorsement by ACOG helped to increase the utilization of antenatal corticosteroids dramatically.[11] Within a few years, 70% to 90% of women who delivered at less than 34 weeks had received a course of corticosteroids.[12] In fact the logo for the Cochrane Collaboration features one of the forest plots from the Crowley meta-analysis because of the tremendous impact of this study on obstetric practice and outcomes for premature infants.

Subgroup analysis from the initial trial on antenatal corticosteroids suggested that effectiveness peaked between 2 and 7 days from the initial injection.[5] This led to the phenomenon of mothers being considered "steroid complete" at 48 hours. Subsequent systematic reviews also suggested a waning of steroid effect at 7 days, prompting concern about the management of mothers who remained pregnant after 7 days but were still at high risk for preterm delivery and adverse neonatal outcomes. Hence the third conclusion in the history of corticosteroids: Clinicians can become overeager in the use of certain interventions before there are adequate supportive data. The administration of repeat courses of corticosteroids to pregnant women at risk for preterm delivery quickly became common practice in the 1990s. In a 1995 survey of perinatologists, 96% of respondents reported willingness to administer more than one course, and more than half would give four or more repeat courses.[13] The routine use of repeat corticosteroids became so widespread that the NIH reconvened a consensus conference in 2000, only 6 years after the conference to promote corticosteroid adoption, to address this issue.[14] The panel recommended that repeat courses of corticosteroids be limited to patient participating in RCTs, because of the insufficient data on the safety and efficacy of this practice.

It is also interesting to note how arbitrary choices can insinuate themselves into standard clinical practice. The initial Liggins and Howie trial used betamethasone as a 1:1 mixture of betamethasone phosphate and betamethasone acetate (currently available as Celestone), as have nearly all subsequent trials.[5] The two injection course of 12 mg given at a 24-hour interval was also empirically chosen by Liggins and Howie.[5] Despite clear evidence of the effectiveness of this therapy, this dosage and this regimen have never been rigorously tested in clinical studies. In fact, this regimen has become such a standard practice that future clinical trials to test them will be difficult, or even impossible to conduct.

This article takes a critical look at the evidence for the efficacy and safety of antenatal corticosteroids that has accumulated over the past 40 years. The story of antenatal corticosteroids is ongoing, and there is much at stake as we continue to perfect the use of this vital therapy.

EFFICACY OF ANTENATAL CORTICOSTEROID TREATMENT

The most recent Cochrane review on antenatal corticosteroids for women at risk for preterm birth included 21 studies of 3885 patients and 4269 infants.[15] The authors included all randomized comparisons of antenatal corticosteroid (betamethasone, dexamethasone, or hydrocortisone) administration to placebo or no treatment for women expected to deliver preterm. Treatment with a single course of antenatal corticosteroids decreased the risk of neonatal death by 31% (95% confidence interval [CI] 19%–42%, 3956 infants). The risk of RDS was reduced by 34% (95% CI 27%–41%, 4038 infants), IVH by 46% (95% CI 31%–57%, 2872 infants), NEC by 54% (95% CI 26%–71%, 1675 infants), and infection in the first 48 hours by 44% (95% CI 15%–62%, 1319 infants). Need for respiratory support and admission to the neonatal intensive care unit were also reduced by therapy.

In studies that examined long-term outcomes of antenatal corticosteroids, treatment was associated with a 51% reduction in developmental delay in childhood (95% CI 0–76%, 518 children) and a trend toward fewer children having cerebral palsy (relative risk [RR] 0.60, 95% CI 0.34–1.03, 904 children). The longest specified duration of follow-up in these studies was 6 years.

The authors concluded that a single course of antenatal corticosteroids should be considered routine for preterm delivery. In fact the weight of this evidence was so compelling that "There is no need for further trials of a single course of antenatal corticosteroids versus placebo in singleton pregnancies."[15(p14)]

EFFICACY IN SPECIAL PATIENT POPULATIONS

Though the efficacy of antenatal corticosteroids to improve outcomes after preterm birth may be established for singleton infants, there remain questions about efficacy in specific patient populations.

Multiple Gestations

Patients with multiple gestations are at significantly higher risk of delivering preterm. In 2008, 58.9% of twins were delivered preterm (<37 weeks' gestation), with 11.6% of them born before 32 weeks.[16] In contrast, only 10.6% of singletons were born preterm, with 1.6% born before 32 weeks.[16] Triplet gestations and higher order multiples are at even higher risk. Patients with multiple gestations are more likely to be delivered preterm for a multitude of reasons, including higher rates of obstetric complications such as preterm labor and preterm rupture of membranes, and the increased incidence of maternal complications such as preeclampsia in these pregnancies.

In the most recent Cochrane review, antenatal corticosteroids were not effective in reducing the risk of RDS, IVH, or neonatal death for women with multiple pregnancies.[15] In a much larger population-based study examining the incidence of RDS in singleton, twin and triplet gestations exposed to antenatal corticosteroids, Blickstein and colleagues demonstrated that plurality is an effect modifier.[17] However, in this study a complete course of antenatal corticosteroids did reduce the risk of RDS compared to no steroid treatment in both twin and triplet pregnancies. Smaller, retrospective studies have been divided on the effectiveness of antenatal corticosteroids to reduce neonatal morbidity and mortality in preterm twin versus singleton pregnancies.[18,19]

There may be physiologic reasons for the diminished effectiveness of antenatal corticosteroids in multiple gestations. Some authors have suggested that the larger volume of distribution in the maternal and fetal compartments in multiple gestations would have a dilutional effect on the concentrations of drugs reaching the fetuses.[20] However, one study of the pharmacodynamics of betamethasone showed that the volume of distribution was actually the same between singleton and twin pregnancies.[21] These investigators did demonstrate that twin pregnancies exhibited a shorter half-life and faster clearance of betamethasone, which they postulated was an effect of the two fetoplacental units accelerated metabolism of betamethasone, which could potentially decrease effectiveness. More recently Gyamfi and colleagues demonstrated that maternal and umbilical cord serum betamethasone concentrations at delivery did not differ between singleton and twin gestations, suggesting that any apparent decrease in effectiveness of steroids in twin pregnancies is not due to inadequate fetal drug levels.[22] This analysis was restricted to patients receiving multiple courses of antenatal corticosteroids who delivered within 1 week of betamethasone administration.

The most current evidence does not confirm the efficacy of antenatal corticosteroids in multiple gestations. Yet guidelines uniformly advocate for corticosteroid administration in these pregnancies at risk for preterm birth because of the weight of the evidence in singleton gestations. The most likely reason that studies in multiple gestations have not demonstrated efficacy is the quality of the available data, which do not include large prospective trials comparing corticosteroid treatment versus no treatment. Only two prospective trials totaling 167 twins and 157 controls supplied the data for the Cochrane review. The remainder of the evidence comes from retrospective studies with multiple potential confounders. The Cochrane authors suggested that there may be additional unpublished data on twin pregnancies that may help clarify the benefit of treatment in this population, as further trials will be difficult to conduct.

Obese Women

The problem of obesity has reached epidemic proportions across developed nations and even across the globe.[23] Obesity is an independent risk factor for many different adverse obstetric outcomes, although most studies have not found a strong association between obesity and spontaneous preterm delivery.[24,25] Still, with the high prevalence of obesity, the need for administration of antenatal corticosteroids to an obese patient is a common occurrence in obstetric practice. Just as in multiple gestations, it has been hypothesized that obesity might influence the effectiveness of antenatal corticosteroids because of differences in tissue distribution and drug elimination. However, Hashima and colleagues found that body mass index (BMI) did not influence neonatal outcome in women receiving a single course of antenatal corticosteroids.[26] In fact, in a study of maternal and cord serum betamethasone levels, there was no significant difference between obese and nonobese women (BMI $\geq$30 kg/m^2 vs BMI $\leq$30 kg/m^2) after controlling for confounding factors.[22] Therefore, despite theoretical concerns, there is no current evidence supporting an alternative antenatal corticosteroid regimen based upon maternal BMI.

Intrauterine Fetal Growth Restriction

The literature appears to be conflicting on the efficacy of antenatal corticosteroids for pregnancies complicated by fetal growth restriction. As with the patient populations previously discussed, there are no randomized studies specifically designed to determine the benefits and risks of antenatal corticosteroid treatment in this group and therefore the evidence consists of observational and retrospective trials with their inherent limitations. Largely because the first trial of Liggins and Howie suggested an increased risk of fetal death in pregnancies complicated by hypertension and fetal growth disorders, these patients have been excluded from most of the subsequent trials.[5]

One large population-based study of infants with intrauterine growth restriction (IUGR) demonstrated that the benefits of antenatal corticosteroids were similar to those seen in normally grown infants. This study included 1720 infants between 25 and 30 weeks' gestation with outcomes reported in the Vermont Oxford Network database.[27] The risks of RDS, IVH, and neonatal death were all significantly reduced by therapy. Among the outcomes evaluated, only necrotizing enterocolitis was not reduced in neonates with IUGR. Interestingly, there was a smaller reduction in the rate of RDS among IUGR infants (odds ratio [OR] 0.70) than normally grown infants (OR 0.50). This information seems to refute the premise that in utero "stress" causes the release of endogenous steroid hormones, which negates the effect of exogenous treatment, though the magnitude of the corticosteroid effect might be less in growth-restricted infants because of this phenomenon. Another case control study looked at long-term outcomes of preterm infants with growth restriction secondary to placental insufficiency.[28] Of 124 infants born between 26 and 32 weeks' gestation survival without disability or handicap at 2 years of age was higher in the corticosteroid group than in matched controls. Conversely, a recent systematic review of antenatal corticosteroid therapy for growth-restricted, preterm infants concluded that treatment has no effect on neonatal morbidity or mortality in this population.[29]

Not only is there a degree of uncertainty about efficacy of antenatal corticosteroids for growth-restricted fetuses, but also there is some concern about the safety of use in this population. IUGR is associated with alterations in cardiovascular function to maintain adequate blood flow to vital organs. Glucocorticoids are powerful regulators of vascular tone, and it is possible that this has a particularly detrimental effect on brain development and long-term function. In a compelling study using a sheep model, Miller and colleagues demonstrated that IUGR fetuses display significant carotid blood flow reperfusion in response to maternal betamethasone administration, which may lead to lipid peroxidation in the fetal brain, thereby contributing to an increased incidence of cell death.[30] There may also be adverse effects of corticosteroid administration on placental function and fetoplacental dynamics, which place these fetuses at risk for adverse neurological outcomes.[31]

Several investigators have advocated for a RCT to examine whether treatment is truly beneficial for IUGR fetuses.[29,31] This would appear to be particularly prudent given the concerns regarding short- and long-term safety in this population.

Very Early Preterm

Advances in neonatology and obstetric care in the last few decades have resulted in increased survival of extremely premature infants. Because of this, resuscitation of preterm infants before 24 weeks' gestation has become increasingly common. The administration of antenatal corticosteroids at 23 weeks' gestation and even earlier has become more frequent, without clear evidence to support the benefit in this population.

In a post hoc analysis, the Cochrane review evaluated outcomes of antenatal corticosteroid treatment versus placebo by gestational age at entry to the trial.[15] Neonatal death was significantly reduced in corticosteroid-treated infants entering a trial, from 26 to 29 6/7 weeks (RR 0.67, 95% CI 0.45–0.99) but not from less than 26 weeks (RR 1.87, 95% CI 0.61–5.87). Similarly, RDS was reduced in all gestational ages with the exception of less than 26 weeks' gestation. Unfortunately there are very few trials that included pregnancies less than 26 weeks' gestation; only one study with fewer than 30 infants supplied the data for this group.

In 2011, Onland and colleagues published an updated systematic review of RCTs on the effects of antenatal corticosteroids given before 26 weeks' gestation.[32] Nine trials that together randomized 1118 subjects were included; publication dates ranged from 1980 to 2006. Although none of the existing trials actually reported the outcomes in this particular subgroup, metaregression and subgroup meta-analysis revealed no significant reduction of neonatal mortality or morbidity in the corticosteroid-treated group compared with the untreated group. Certainly these analyses may be underpowered to demonstrate effectiveness. It is also possible that antenatal corticosteroids can improve lung function only once adequate numbers of primitive alveoli and lamellar bodies have started to appear, which typically occurs in the saccular phase of lung development beginning at approximately 25 weeks' gestation, though some in vitro studies would suggest a maturational effect can occur earlier in gestation.[33]

However, if there is a beneficial effect of antenatal corticosteroids at very early gestational ages, it may be more evident in mortality rates and neurologic morbidity than in prevention of RDS. Evidence from the EPICure study, a prospective cohort study of all infants born at less than 26 weeks' gestation in the United Kingdom and Ireland in 1995, showed that exposed newborns had decreased rates of death (OR 0.57, 95% CI 0.37–0.85) and severe IVH (OR 0.39, 95% CI 0.22–0.77), but not a decreased rate of RDS.[34] A more recent retrospective cohort study of 181 infants born at 23 weeks' gestation also showed that antenatal corticosteroids decreased the risk of death (OR 0.32, 95% CI 0.12–0.84) relative to unexposed infants.[35] A retrospective series from Japan even demonstrated a decrease in mortality of infants born at 22 or 23 weeks' gestation after exposure to corticosteroids.[36]

Although the results of observational cohort studies and retrospective analyses are sensitive to various biases, at times they represent the best of our understanding of the evidence, particularly when randomized studies are unavailable. In a large prospective cohort of 4446 infants born at 22 to 25 weeks' gestation published by Tyson and colleagues from the Neonatal Research Network of the National Institute of Child Health and Human Development, multivariable analyses showed that those who received intensive care, were exposed to antenatal corticosteroids, were of female sex, and were from singleton pregnancies and of higher birth weight had reduced rates of death.[37] In addition, among survivors the risk of death or impairment at 18 to 22 months corrected age was also reduced by corticosteroid exposure. Long-term data from the EPICure investigators also showed that antenatal cortico-steroids were associated with an increased mental development index assessed at 2.5 and 6 years of age.[38]

The decisions surrounding the "threshold of viability" are exceedingly difficult, on the part of patients, families, obstetricians, and neonatologists. Even with the most aggressive intervention, the neonatal mortality rate is high, as is the chance of adverse long-term neurodevelopmental outcome. Despite the lack of randomized data on efficacy in the very preterm period, the suggestion of benefit for these preterm infants seems sufficient to recommend its use.

Late Preterm

Most studies to date have evaluated antenatal corticosteroid administration to patients at risk for preterm birth less than 34 0/7 weeks' gestation. Certainly the risk of neonatal death in the late preterm period (34 0/7–36 6/7 weeks) is exceedingly low, and the risk of the major morbidities that antenatal corticosteroid use has been shown to decrease (RDS, IVH, NEC) are relatively rare. However, in deciding whether antenatal corticosteroid use is appropriate at a specific gestational age, the frequency of disease must be balanced by the total number of infants who may benefit. In fact, because nearly 75% of all preterm births occur in the late preterm period, the absolute number of infants being admitted to the neonatal intensive care unit for respiratory distress or a respiratory indication is significant.[16]

Interestingly, the Cochrane review supports use of antenatal corticosteroids for women at risk of preterm birth up to 34 6/7 weeks' gestation.[15] This recommendation arose from the apparent decrease in the rate of RDS in the subgroup of infants receiving treatment between 33 and 34 6/7 weeks (RR 0.53, 95% CI 0.31–0.91). The Royal College of Obstetricians and Gynaecologists (RCOG) recommends that clinicians offer a single course of antenatal corticosteroids to women up to 34 6/7 weeks who are at risk of preterm birth.[39]

It is obvious that if antenatal corticosteroids work to improve respiratory function, there is likely to be a continuum of benefit across the preterm, and potentially even the early term period. It has been hypothesized that corticosteroids may be effective at later gestational ages, not because of an increase in surfactant production from type II alveolar cells or acceleration in lung structural development reducing the incidence of classic RDS, but by increasing expression of epithelial sodium channels (ENaCs) that allow the alveoli to convert from active fluid secretion to sodium and fluid absorption with subsequent reduction of fetal lung fluid.

To answer this question formally, the Maternal Fetal Medicine Units Network is currently conducting a prospective, RCT of antenatal corticosteroids for patients at risk for late preterm birth. The trial is expected to be completed in 2014. It will be particularly interesting to see if antenatal corticosteroids confer an overall benefit in this population, or if the benefit is dependent on mode and circumstances of delivery such as cesarean versus vaginal delivery or indicated preterm birth versus spontaneous preterm birth. Multiple studies have suggested the potential benefit of antenatal corticosteroids to decrease respiratory morbidity even at term for patients delivered by elective cesarean.[40–42]

SAFETY OF ANTENATAL CORTICOSTEROID TREATMENT

A single course of antenatal corticosteroids is not associated with any significant short-term fetal or neonatal adverse effects. Specifically, studies have shown no difference in the rate of fetal death in exposed versus unexposed.[15] For the neonate, there is no impact of antenatal corticosteroids on birthweight, hypothalamic–pituitary axis function, or the incidence of proven infection while in the intensive care unit.[15] Importantly, long-term follow-up of those enrolled in RCTs through early adulthood shows no apparent adverse neurologic or cognitive effects from a single course of treatment.[43,44]

There have been no reports of serious maternal complications linked to antenatal corticosteroid treatment. The Cochrane review did not demonstrate any statistically significant difference in the rate of chorioamnionitis (RR 0.91, 95% CI 0.70–1.18) or puerperal sepsis (RR 1.35, 95% CI 0.93–1.95) in treated versus untreated patients.[15] Patients with pregestational or gestational diabetes will frequently experience an increase in hyperglycemia and those on medical treatment may require temporary adjustments in their regimens. For patients with poor glycemic control, inpatient observation during antenatal corticosteroid treatment may be required. Of note, patients with diabetes have universally been excluded from RCTs on antenatal corticosteroids, so the benefit of corticosteroid treatment has been extrapolated from the nondiabetic population.

There are no specific contraindications to a single course of antenatal corticosteroids. However, there is concern that the immunosuppressive effect would exacerbate systemic infection or activate latent disease. Active tuberculosis has been suggested as a potential contraindication for antenatal corticosteroid treatment, although there is no evidence upon which this is based. Clearly this will not be as common a problem in developed countries as it will be in developing countries where antenatal corticosteroid administration is still a rare practice.[45] Close monitoring of the safety of corticosteroid treatment in developing countries as the use increases is critical.

Preterm Premature Rupture of Membranes

Data from the Cochrane review demonstrates reductions in neonatal death, RDS, IVH, and NEC in the subgroup of infants whose mothers received antenatal corticosteroids for preterm premature rupture of membranes (PPROM).[15] There is no increase in maternal or neonatal infection in this setting. However, concern remains about use of corticosteroids in this population because of the increased risk of chorioamnionitis and the strong association between clinical chorioamnionitis and cystic periventricular leukomalacia as well as cerebral palsy.[46] A recent meta-analysis of observational studies demonstrated that antenatal corticosteroids were effective in reducing neonatal mortality and morbidity (to include severe IVH and periventricular leukomalacia) in the setting of both histologic and clinical chorioamnionitis. However, because of lingering concern about the preterm delivery in the setting of chorioamnionitis largely stemming from a trial of weekly antenatal corticosteroids, ACOG still does not fully endorse corticosteroid administration after 32 weeks' gestation.[47,48]

Certainly the etiology of periventricular leukomalacia and cerebral palsy after preterm birth is an active area of investigation. Infection and inflammation are believed to be important pathophysiologic factors. At this time we can certainly recommend that delivery not be delayed in the setting of clinical chorioamnionitis for administration of antenatal corticosteroids. But the evidence overall supports administration of antenatal corticosteroids for patients with PPROM up to 32 to 34 weeks in the absence of overt infection.

CHOICE OF ANTENATAL CORTICOSTEROID

Both betamethasone and dexamethasone have demonstrated efficacy in the promotion of fetal maturity. Betamethasone (given as a combination of betamethasone sodium phosphate and betamethasone acetate) is administered as two doses of 12 mg given intramuscularly, 24 hours apart. Dexamethasone sodium phosphate is administered as four doses of 6 mg given intramuscularly, 12 hours apart. These agents are structurally similar, fluorinated compounds with minimal mineralocorticoid activity and weak immunosuppressive activity with short-term administration. However, a betamethasone suspension (Celestone Soluspan) frequently used in this country has a longer half-life because of the prolonged absorption of the betamethasone acetate component. In addition, although they have comparable genomic potencies because of similar high affinities for the glucocorticoid receptor, the nongenomic effects of dexamethasone appear to be significantly stronger.[49] The bottom line is that these are different drugs, and it should come as no great surprise if they have different effects.

In a subgroup analysis of antenatal corticosteroids versus placebo or no treatment by type of corticosteroid, Roberts and Dalziel found that betamethasone treatment resulted in a greater reduction in RDS than dexamethasone treatment (RR 0.56, 95% CI 0.68–0.93).[15] There were no other statistically significant differences between groups, except that dexamethasone significantly increased the incidence of puerperal sepsis. This indirect comparison would seem to favor betamethasone administration. However, a subsequent Cochrane review summarized the evidence from trials, which directly compared these two agents.[50] This analysis demonstrated that dexamethasone decreased the risk of IVH compared with betamethasone (RR 0.44, 95% CI 0.21–0.92). No difference was seen for any other outcomes evaluated, including severe IVH.

In a large historical cohort study from the National Institute of Child Health and Human Development (NICHD) Neonatal Research Network Registry, Lee and colleagues reported on the outcomes of very low birthweight infants (401–1500 g) exposed to betamethasone, dexamethasone, or no corticosteroid treatment.[51] Betamethasone was associated with a significantly reduced risk for neonatal death. In addition, there were trends of decreased risk for other adverse neonatal outcomes with exposure to betamethasone over dexamethasone. These authors concluded that "it may be in the best interests of neonates to receive betamethasone rather than dexamethasone when available."[51(p1503)]

Yet in a recent RCT comparing betamethasone to dexamethasone there was no difference seen in neonatal mortality, RDS, NEC or sepsis.[52] However, neonates exposed to betamethasone had a significantly higher rate of IVH (17% vs 5.7%). It would appear that the randomized data tends to favor dexamethasone over betamethasone because of this reduction in IVH. However, the conclusions are clearly inconsistent across the range of studies. Importantly, there are no long-term outcome data on safety or efficacy for those treated with dexamethasone as there is with betamethasone. Additional RCTs are necessary to determine the preferable agent as well as to establish the optimal treatment regimen. According to ACOG guidelines, both betamethasone and dexamethasone are acceptable for promotion of fetal maturity in women at risk for preterm delivery.

TIMING OF EFFECTIVENESS

After reviewing the available evidence, the 1994 NIH consensus panel concluded that the optimal benefit of antenatal corticosteroids was seen at 24 hours to 7 days after initiation of treatment. The panel recommended that further studies were necessary to determine whether the beneficial effects diminished after 7 days and whether retreatment at some time point would be necessary.

In the subgroup analysis of antenatal corticosteroids versus placebo or no treatment by entry to delivery interval, the Cochrane analysis demonstrated a reduction in the risk of RDS in treated infants born before 48 hours (RR 0.63, 95% CI 0.43–0.93) and between 1 and 7 days after treatment (RR 0.46, 95% CI 0.35–0.60) but not those born before 24 hours or after 7 days.[15] Curiously, neonatal death was reduced in treated infants born before 24 hours (RR 0.53, 95% CI 0.29–0.96) and before 48 hours (RR 0.49, 95% CI 0.30–0.81) but *not* those born between 1 and 7 days after treatment or after 7 days. IVH was reduced in those born before 48 hours but not in any other time period studied.

Additional studies have attempted to clarify the duration of corticosteroid effectiveness. Vermillion and colleagues published a retrospective analysis of neonates treated with antenatal corticosteroids who were delivered between 28 and 34 weeks' gestation.[53] They found no difference between those delivered 8 to 14 days after treatment compared to those delivered within 7 days. Peaceman and colleagues also found no difference in outcomes of those delivered more than 7 days after treatment compared to those delivered within 7 days, in a study of 197 neonates whose mothers received a complete single course of antenatal corticosteroids.[54]

Even if there is some decline in the effectiveness of antenatal corticosteroids over time, it is likely that this decline is not static across all gestational ages or birthweights. There may be a relationship between the specific gestational age at administration and the gestational age at delivery. Ring and colleagues reported on the outcomes of 357 singleton pregnancies delivered between 26 and 34 weeks after completing a single course of antenatal corticosteroids.[55] Neonatal outcomes were compared between those exposed within 14 days of delivery and those exposed after 14 days. Outcomes among treatment groups were stratified by gestational age at delivery (<28 weeks, ≥28 weeks). A steroid-to-delivery interval of more than 14 days was associated with an increased need for ventilatory support and surfactant use, particularly for those delivered beyond 28 weeks.

In an intriguing article published in 2007, Simon Gates and Peter Brocklehurst criticized the subgroup analyses published in the systematic reviews on antenatal corticosteroids that led to the conclusion that effectiveness declines after 7 days.[56] They cited four ways in which the data—and therefore the conclusion—could be unsound. The first problem listed was the arbitrary choice of 24 hours and 7 days as the cutoff points for the subgroups, which the first clinical trial and most subsequent trials have analyzed. Unfortunately, this means that all infants born at term will be in the more than 7 days subgroup; because of a lower incidence of adverse outcomes in these patients it is unlikely that a statistically significant difference would be found. This does not equate to a complete lack of treatment effectiveness at 8 days, although that has been a frequent conclusion. Gates and Brocklehurst also pointed out that statistical tests of interaction should be used to assess subgroup differences, not tests of statistical significance, because subgroups with fewer trials are less likely to give significant results even if their effects are the same. Finally, subgroup analyses classified by variables that arise after randomization have a high risk of producing misleading results because of bias. Differences in effectiveness of the intervention may arise because of differences in the subgroup.

Without knowing the exact time course of effectiveness, it is difficult to know if and when repeat or rescue courses of antenatal corticosteroids are necessary. This clinical dilemma is further complicated by the difficulty in predicting who will have a preterm delivery and when that delivery will occur. In a recent study in Ireland, the ratio of women given a complete course of corticosteroids to the number who actually delivered before 34 weeks' gestation was 4:1.[57] Analysis by indication for preterm birth revealed this ratio to be 15:1 in suspected preterm labor, 8:1 in antepartum hemorrhage, and 2:1 in both PPROM and medically indicated preterm birth. McLaughlin and colleagues also looked at the accuracy of physicians in timing the administration of antenatal corticosteroids.[58] Overall, women treated before 28 weeks' gestation were more likely to give birth more than 7 days later than those treated after 28 weeks. It is difficult to say if those data reflect a quicker tendency by physicians to treat patients at risk of preterm birth at earlier gestations for fear of adverse neonatal outcomes, or an actual difference in likelihood to deliver between these groups. Women who received antenatal corticosteroids because of placenta previa, multiple gestation, or cervical incompetence were more likely to remain pregnant in this study, while those with hypertension or idiopathic preterm labor had a higher rate of delivery within 7 days.

TIMING OF ADMINISTRATION
Multiple Courses

Over the last decade, a number of multicenter, prospective trials comparing a single course of antenatal corticosteroid treatment to multiple courses have been published.[59–61] The results of 10 RCTs, involving 4730 women and 5650 neonates, have been summarized recently in a Cochrane review.[62] Treatment of women who remained at risk of preterm birth 7 or more days after an initial course of antenatal corticosteroids with repeat dose(s) compared with no repeat treatment reduced the risk of infant respiratory distress syndrome (RR 0.83, 95% CI 0.75–0.91). In addition, serious infant morbidity was reduced by repeat dose(s) (RR 0.84, 95% CI 0.75–0.94). Serious infant morbidity was variously defined by the trialists but generally included a composite of death, RDS, severe IVH, PVL, and NEC. Treatment with repeat dose(s) was associated with a reduction in mean birthweight (mean difference –75.79 g, 95% CI –117.63 to 33.96).

Four of the trials included in the Cochrane analysis reported data from early childhood follow-up. No statistically significant differences were seen for children in the repeat corticosteroid group as compared to controls. Outcomes examined included death to early childhood follow-up, survival free of any disability, survival free of any major disability, and composite serious outcome at childhood follow-up.

The authors concluded that short-term benefits support the use of repeat dose(s) of antenatal corticosteroids for women who have received an initial course and remain at risk for preterm birth 7 or more days later. However, they noted that although limited evidence from early childhood shows no evidence of harm, there is no proof of long-term benefit either. In addition, there are no data on overall health, neurodevelopment, and cardiovascular and metabolic function later in childhood or in adulthood after exposure to repeat dose(s).

Although overall there was no difference in outcomes assessed in early childhood across the studies, in the MFMU Network trial six children were diagnosed with cerebral palsy in the repeat corticosteroid group whereas only one child was diagnosed with cerebral palsy in the control group. All had received four or more courses of antenatal corticosteroids, five were born at 34 or more weeks of gestation, and none of the pregnancies had obvious perinatal complications. Though this difference did not reach statistical significance, the striking nature of this finding would suggest caution in prescribing multiple courses of antenatal corticosteroids.

Rescue Course

One strategy, which seems to have come into wide clinical use, again with a paucity of supporting data, is to administer a "rescue" course of antenatal corticosteroids. Patients who have received an initial course of antenatal corticosteroids but do not deliver within 7 to 14 days may receive one repeat corticosteroid course known as the "rescue" course. Of course, given the limitations in the data on the timing of effectiveness of corticosteroids, it is not clear if it is appropriate to give this rescue course after 7 days, 14 days, or longer. It is also not clear if this interval should change depending on the timing of the initial course or if the rescue course should be given routinely or only if preterm birth is again deemed "imminent." It seems obvious that the same issues with timing the rescue course will arise as with the initial one.

However, there is increasing data that the rescue approach might be both effective and safe. Vermillion and colleagues published a retrospective cohort study of 152 women at risk for preterm delivery who received a corticosteroid course before 28 weeks.[63] Outcomes were compared for women readmitted for preterm labor after 28 weeks who received a single rescue dose of corticosteroid versus those who did not. Rescue corticosteroid administration was significantly associated with a reduction in frequency of RDS as well as mean days on the ventilator. Multiple logistic regression confirmed that the rescue dose was independently associated with a reduction in the rate of RDS. More recently, Garite and colleagues published the results of a randomized trial with a rescue approach.[64] Patients with singleton or twin pregnancies less than 33 weeks, who had received a single course of antenatal corticosteroids before 30 weeks and were at risk for preterm delivery in the next week, were enrolled. Patients were randomized to a single rescue course of betamethasone or placebo. The treatment group had reduced composite morbidity (OR 0.65, 95% CI 0.44–0.97) as well as a reduced frequency of RDS (OR 0.64, 95% CI 0.43–0.95). Treatment did not decrease mean birthweight or impact the rate of IUGR.

GUIDELINES BY MAJOR SOCIETIES

In February of 2011, ACOG published a new Committee Opinion on antenatal corticosteroid therapy for fetal maturation.[65] The College reaffirmed its support for administration of a single course of antenatal corticosteroids to pregnant women between 24 and 34 weeks' gestation at risk of preterm delivery within 7 days. They do not recommend administering antenatal corticosteroids before 24 weeks' gestation because of sparse evidence in this population. Also, in a departure from earlier publications, ACOG supports a single rescue course of antenatal corticosteroids under the following circumstances: if the antecedent treatment was given more than 2 weeks prior, if the gestational age is less than 32 6/7 weeks, and if the patient is deemed likely to give birth within the next week (rather than a scheduled administration).

The most recent RCOG guidelines differ from those of ACOG in a few interesting ways. The Royal College supports administration of a single course of antenatal corticosteroids between 24 0/7 weeks and 34 6/7 weeks, the upper limit arising from the Cochrane data presented earlier. However, they state that antenatal corticosteroids can be considered for women between 23 0/7 weeks and 23 6/7 weeks who are at risk of preterm birth, as long as this decision is "made at a senior level taking all clinical aspects into consideration."[39(p3)] In addition, the RCOG recommends that antenatal corticosteroids should be given to all patients for whom an elective cesarean is planned prior to 38 6/7 weeks, largely based on the results of one randomized trial of betamethasone versus no treatment that decreased the rate of admission for RDS.[66] In the RCOG guideline, rescue corticosteroids "should only be considered with caution in those pregnancies where the first course was given at less than 26 0/7 weeks of gestation and another obstetric indication arises later in pregnancy."[39(p17)]

Although each of these guidelines appear reasonable, it is clear from the data already presented that these recommendations stem from varying interpretations of the data rather than comprehensively studied protocols.

FUTURE RESEARCH

Throughout this article the limitations in the current evidence on the safety and efficacy of antenatal corticosteroids have been highlighted. Although the evidence for benefit of a single course of antenatal corticosteroids for women at risk of preterm birth between 24 and 34 weeks is clear, questions remain about the best dose, best corticosteroid, length of effectiveness, as well as need for and timing of repeat corticosteroids. There are limitations in the evidence for all of the specific patient populations mentioned. Additional RCTs would be welcome. But even without regard to the time and expense required for randomized studies, because of the routine use of antenatal corticosteroids in these populations already, such trials will be exceedingly difficult to conduct.

To address some of these questions without new trials, a group of investigators representing each of the major trials of repeat dosing have been funded to conduct an individual patient data meta-analysis. Led by Caroline Crowther of the University of Adelaide, the primary goal of this study is to determine the efficacy and safety of various repeat dosing approaches. Hopefully this will be able to answer other outstanding questions regarding corticosteroids in lieu of additional studies.

SUMMARY

Though the preterm birth rate in the United States has finally begun to decline, preterm birth remains a critical public health problem. The administration of antenatal corticosteroids to improve outcomes after preterm birth is one of the most important interventions in obstetrics. This article summarizes the evidence for antenatal corticosteroid efficacy and safety that has accumulated since Graham Liggins and Ross Howie first introduced this therapy. Although antenatal corticosteroids have proven effective for singleton pregnancies at risk for preterm birth between 26 and 34 weeks' gestation, questions remain about the utility in specific patient populations such as multiple gestations, very early preterm gestations, and pregnancies complicated by IUGR. In addition, there is still uncertainty about the length of corticosteroid effectiveness and the need for repeat or rescue courses. Though a significant amount of data has accumulated on antenatal corticosteroids over the past 40 years, more information is still needed to refine the use of this therapy and improve outcomes for these at-risk patients.

REFERENCES

1. Martin JA, Hamilton BE, Sutton PD. Births: final data for 2006. Natl Vit Stat Rep 2009;57:1–104.
2. Hamilton BE, Martin JA, Ventura SJ. Births: preliminary data for 2009. Natl Vit Stat Rep 2010;59:1–19.

3. Martin JA, Osterman MJK, Sutton PD. Are preterm births on the decline in the United States? Recent data from the National Vital Statistics System. NCHS Data Brief 2010;39:1–8.
4. Liggins GC. Premature delivery of foetal lambs infused with glucocorticoids. J Endocrinol 1969;45:515–23.
5. Liggins GC, Howie RN. A controlled trial of antepartum glucocorticoid treatment for prevention of the respiratory distress syndrome in premature infants. Pediatrics 1972;50:515–25.
6. Villee CA, Villee DB, Zuckerman J. Respiratory distress syndrome. New York: Academic Press; 1973.
7. Leviton LC, Baker S, Hassol A, et al. An exploration of opinion and practice patterns affecting low use of antenatal corticosteroids. Am J Obstet Gynecol 1995;173:312–6.
8. Bronstein JM, Goldenberg RL. Practice variation in the use of corticosteroids: a comparison of eight data sets. Am J Obstet Gynecol 1995;173:296–8.
9. Crowley P, Chalmers I, Kierse MJ. The effects of corticosteroid administration before preterm delivery: an overview of the evidence from controlled trials. BJOG 1990;97: 11–25.
10. NIH Consensus Development Panel on the effect of corticosteroids for fetal maturation on perinatal outcomes. JAMA 1995;273:413–8.
11. ACOG Committee Opinion. Antenatal corticosteroid therapy for fetal maturation. Int J Gynaecol Obstet 1995;48:340–2.
12. Leviton LC, Goldenberg RL, Baker CS, et al. Methods to encourage the use of antenatal corticosteroid therapy for fetal maturation: a randomized controlled trial. JAMA 1999;281:46–52.
13. Planer BC, Ballard RA, Ballard PL, et al. Antenatal corticosteroid (ANCS) use in preterm labor in the USA. Pediatr Res 1996;39:110A.
14. NIH Consensus Development Panel. Antenatal corticosteroids revisited: repeat courses. Obstet Gynecol 2000;98:144–50.
15. Roberts D, Dalziel S. Antenatal corticosteroids for accelerating fetal lung maturation for women at risk of preterm birth. Cochrane Database Syst Rev 2006;3:CD004454.
16. Martin JA, Hamilton BE, Sutton PD, et al. Births: final data for 2008. Natl Vit Stat Rep 2010;59:1–72.
17. Blickstein I, Shinwell E, Lusky A, et al. Plurality-dependent risk of respiratory distress syndrome among very-low-birthweight infants and antepartum corticosteroid treatment. Am J Obstet Gynecol 2005;192:360–4.
18. Batista L, Winovitch KC, Rumney PJ, et al. A case-control comparison of the effectiveness of betamethasone to prevent neonatal morbidity and mortality in preterm twin and singleton pregnancies. Am J Perinatol 2008;25:449–53.
19. Choi SJ, Song SE, Seo ES, et al. The effect of single or multiple courses of antenatal corticosteroid therapy on neonatal respiratory distress syndrome in singleton versus twin pregnancies. Aust NZ Obstet Gynaecol 2009;49:173–9.
20. Quist-Therson EC, Myhr TL, Ohlsson A. Antenatal steroids to prevent respiratory distress syndrome: multiple gestation as an effect modifier. Acta Obstet Gynecol Scand 1999;78:388–92.
21. Ballabh P, Lo ES, Kumari J, et al. Pharmacokinetics of betamethasone in twin and singleton pregnancy. Clin Pharmacol Ther 2002;71:39–45.
22. Gyamfi C, Mele L, Wapner RJ, et al. The effect of plurality and obesity on betamethasone concentrations in women at risk for preterm delivery. Am J Obstet Gynecol 2010;203:219.e1–5.
23. Chescheir NC. Global obesity and the effect on women's health. Obstet Gynecol 2011;117:1213–22.

24. Weiss JL, Malone FD, Emig D, et al. Obesity, obstetric complications and cesarean delivery rate—a population-based screening study. Am J Obstet Gynecol 2004;190; 1091–7.

25. McDonald SD, Han Z, Mulla S, et al. Overweight and obesity in mothers and risk of preterm birth and low birthweight infants: a systematic review and meta-analysis. BMJ 2010;341:c3428.

26. Hashima JN, Lai Y, Wapner RJ. The effect of body mass index on neonatal outcome in women receiving a single course of antenatal corticosteroids. Am J Obstet Gynecol 2010;202:263.e1–5.

27. Bernstein IM, Horbar JD, Badger GJ, et al. Morbidity and mortality among very-low-birthweight neonates with intrauterine growth restriction. Am J Obstet Gynecol 2000;182:198–206.

28. Schaap AH, Wolf H, Bruinse HW, et al. Effects of antenatal corticosteroid administration on mortality and long-term morbidity in early, preterm, growth-restricted infants. Obstet Gynecol 2001;97:954–60.

29. Torrance HL, Derks JB, Scherion SA, et al. Is antenatal steroid treatment effective in preterm IUGR fetuses? Acta Obstet Gynecol Scand 2009;88:1068–73.

30. Miller SL, Chai M, Loose J, et al. The effects of maternal betamethasone administration on the growth-restricted fetus. Endocrinology 2007;148:1288–95.

31. Vidaeff AC, Blackwell SC. Potential risks and benefits of antenatal corticosteroid therapy prior to preterm birth in pregnancies complicated by fetal growth restriction. Obstet Gynecol Clin North Am 2011;38:205–14.

32. Onland W, de Laat MW, Mol BW, et al. Effects of antenatal corticosteroids given prior to 26' weeks gestation: a systematic review of randomized controlled trials. Am J Perinatol 2011;28:33–44.

33. Gonzales LW, Ballard PL, Ertsey R, et al. Glucocorticoids and thyroid hormones stimulate biochemical and morphological differentiation of human fetal lung in organ culture. J Clin Endocrinol Metab 1986;62:678–91.

34. Costeloe K, Hennessy E, Gibson AT, et al. The EPICure study: outcomes to discharge from hospital for infants born at the threshold of viability. Pediatrics 2000;106:659–71.

35. Hayes EJ, Paul DA, Stahl GE, et al. Effect of antenatal corticosteroids on survival for neonates born at 23 weeks of gestation. Obstet Gynecol 2008;111:921–6.

36. Mori R, Kusada S, Fujimura M, et al. Antenatal corticosteroids promote survival of extremely preterm infants born at 22 to 23 weeks gestation. J Pediatr 2011;110:114.e1.

37. Tyson JE, Parikh NA, Langer J, et al. Intensive care for extreme prematurity—moving beyond gestational age. NEJM 2008;358:1672–81.

38. Costeloe K, EPICure study group. EPICure: facts and figures: why preterm labor should be treated. BJOG 2006;113(Suppl):10–2.

39. Royal College of Obstetricians. Green Top Guideline No 7: Antenatal corticosteroids to reduce neonatal morbidity and mortality. London: Royal College of Obstetricians; 2010.

40. Tita ATN, Landon MB, Spong CY, et al. Timing of elective repeat cesarean at term and neonatal outcomes. N Engl J Med 2009;360:111–20.

41. Hansen AK, Wisborg K, Uldbjerg N, et al. Risk of respiratory morbidity in term infants delivered by elective cesarean section: cohort study. BMJ 2008;336:85–7.

42. Stutchfield P, Whitaker R, Russell I. Antenatal betamethasone and incidence of neonatal respiratory distress after elective cesarean section: a pragmatic randomized trial. BMJ 2005;331:662.

43. Smolders-de Haas H, Neuvel J, Schumand B, et al. Physical development and medical history of children who were treated antenatally with corticosteroids to prevent respiratory distress syndrome: a 10- to 12-year followup. Pediatrics 1990;86: 65–70.

44. Dessens AB, Haas H, Kpooe JG. Twenty-year follow-up of antenatal corticosteroid treatment. Pediatrics 2000;105:e77.

45. Mwansa-Kambafwile J, Cousens S, Hansen T, et al. Antenatal steroids in preterm labor for the prevention of neonatal deaths due to complications of preterm birth. Int J Epidemiol 2010;39 (Suppl):i122–33.

46. Wu YW, Colford JM Jr. Chorioamnionitis as a risk factor for cerebral palsy: a meta-analysis. JAMA 2000;284:1417–24.

47. Lee MJ, Davies J, Guinn D, et al. Single versus weekly courses of antenatal corticosteroids in preterm premature rupture of membranes. Obstet Gynecol 2004;103: 274–81.

48. American College of Obstetricians and Gynecologists (ACOG). Antenatal corticosteroid therapy for fetal maturation. Committee Opinion No. 475. Obstet Gynecol 2011;117:422–4.

49. Buttgereit F, Brand MD, Burmester GR. Equivalent doses and relative drug potencies for non-genomic glucocorticoid effects: a novel glucocorticoid hierarchy. Biochem Pharmacol 1999;58:363–8.

50. Brownfoot FC, Crowther CA, Middleton P. Different corticosteroids and regimens for accelerating fetal lung maturation for women at risk for preterm birth. Cochrane Database Syst Rev 2008;4:CD006764.

51. Lee BH, Stoll BJ, McDonald SA, et al. Adverse neonatal outcomes associated with antenatal dexamethasone versus antenatal betamethasone. Pediatrics 2006;117: 1503–10.

52. Elimian A, Garry D, Figueroa R, et al. Antenatal betamethasone compared with dexamethasone (betacode trial): a randomized controlled trial. Obstet Gynecol 2007; 110:26–30.

53. Vermillion ST, Soper DE, Newman RB. Is betamethasone effective for longer than 7 days after treatment? Obstet Gynecol 2001;97:491–3.

54. Peaceman AM, Bajaj K, Kumar P, et al. The interval between a single course of antenatal steroids and delivery and its association with neonatal outcomes. Am J Obstet Gynecol 2005;193:1165–9.

55. Ring AM, Garland JS, Stafiel BR, et al. The effect of a prolonged time interval between antenatal corticosteroid administration and delivery on outcomes in preterm neonates: a cohort study. Am J Obstet Gynecol 2007;196:457.e1–e6.

56. Gates S, Brocklehurst P. Decline in effectiveness of antenatal corticosteroids with time to real birth: real or artifact? BMJ 2007;335:77–9.

57. Mahony R, McKeating A, Murphy T, et al. Appropriate antenatal corticosteroid use in women at risk for preterm birth before 34 weeks of gestation. BJOG 2010;117:963–7.

58. McLaughlin KJ, Crowther CA, Vigneswaran P, et al. Who remains undelivered more than seven days after a single course of prenatal corticosteroids and gives birth at less than 34 weeks? Aust NZ J Obstet Gynecol 2002;42:353–7.

59. Guinn DA, Atkinson MW, Sillivan L, et al. Single versus weekly courses of antenatal corticosteroids for women at risk of preterm delivery: a randomized controlled trial. JAMA 2001;286:1581–7.

60. Wapner RJ, Sorokin Y, Thom EA, et al. Single versus weekly courses of antenatal corticosteroids: evaluation of safety and efficacy. Am J Obstet Gynecol 2006;195: 633–42.

61. Crowther CA, Haslam RR, Hiller JE, et al. Neonatal respiratory distress syndrome after repeat exposure to antenatal corticosteroids: a randomized controlled trial. Lancet 2006;367:1913–9.

62. Crowther CA, McKinlay CJD, Middleton P, et al. Repeat doses of prenatal cortico-steroids for women at risk for preterm birth for improving neonatal health outcomes. Cochrane Database Syst Rev 2011;6:CD003935.

63. Vermillion ST, Bland ML, Soper DE. Effectiveness of a rescue dose of antenatal betamethasone after an initial single course. Am J Obstet Gynecol 2001;185:1086–9.

64. Garite TJ, Kurtzman J, Maurel K, et al. Impact of a 'rescue course' of antenatal corticosteroids: a multicenter randomized, placebo-controlled trial. Am J Obstet Gynecol 2009;200:248:e1–9.

65. ACOG Committee Opinion. Antenatal corticosteroid therapy for fetal maturation. Obstet Gynecol 2011;117:422–4.

66. Stutchfield P, Whitaker R, Russell I, et al. Antenatal betamethasone and incidence of neonatal respiratory distress after elective cesarean section: pragmatic randomized trial. BMJ 2005;331:662.

Antibiotics in the Management of PROM and Preterm Labor

Brian Mercer, MD[a,b,]*

KEYWORDS

- Antibiotics • Preterm labor • Preterm PROM
- Premature rupture of the membranes

Preterm labor or premature rupture of the membranes (PROM) continue to account for the majority of the nearly 500,000 preterm births that occur in the United States each year,[1] and are of particular importance because of the resultant perinatal morbidity and mortality, and the potential for long-term sequelae in these infants. In many cases, the inciting cause of preterm delivery remains unknown; however, intrauterine infection and inflammation have long been specifically linked to preterm birth, especially that occurring remote from term.[2–5] In both preterm labor and PROM, ascending bacterial colonization of the decidua is believed to be a common inciting event. Unfortunately, strategies to prevent preterm birth through administration of antibiotics to asymptomatic women have met with limited success, and have in some cases led to an increased risk of prematurity.[6–11] Because of this, attention has been given to antibiotic treatment of pregnancies complicated by acute preterm labor or after preterm PROM with the goal of prolonging pregnancy to allow further in utero development of the fetus. In this article, antibiotic therapy as an adjunct to the treatment of preterm labor and PROM for this indication is considered. Although there is considerable overlap between the clinical spectrum of preterm labor and preterm PROM, these entities are considered separately.

ANTIBIOTICS FOR PROM

Fetal membrane rupture before the onset of contractions (premature rupture the membranes, PROM) is responsible for nearly one quarter to one third of preterm births and is associated with brief latency from membrane ruptured to delivery, umbilical cord compression, and an increased risk of chorioamnionitis. It is likely that ascending

The author has nothing to disclose.
[a] Department of Reproductive Biology, Case Western Reserve University, Cleveland, OH, USA
[b] Department of Obstetrics & Maternal-Fetal Medicine, MetroHealth Medical Center, 2500 MetroHealth Drive, Cleveland, OH 44109, USA
* Corresponding author. Department of Obstetrics & Maternal-Fetal Medicine, MetroHealth Medical Center, 2500 MetroHealth Drive, Cleveland, OH 44109.

Obstet Gynecol Clin N Am 39 (2012) 65–76
doi:10.1016/j.ogc.2011.12.007
0889-8545/12/$ – see front matter © 2012 Elsevier Inc. All rights reserved.

bacterial colonization results in local release of proinflammatory cytokines or hydro-lytic enzymes that weaken the fetal membranes some cases. Secondary ascending bacterial colonization of the decidua and amniotic fluid after membrane rupture is also plausible. Amniotic fluid culture and polymerase chain reaction reveal that amniotic fluid collected by amniocentesis from asymptomatic women after preterm PROM will have bacterial colonization in 30% to 50% of samples. Numerous gram-positive, gram-negative, aerobic, and anaerobic species (eg, Bacteroides, Fusobacteria, Peptococcus, Peptostreptococcus, Proprionobacter, Pseudomonas, Staphylococ-cus, and Streptococcus) as well as specific organisms commonly found in the urogenital tract (eg, *Escherichia coli, Enterobacter cloacae, Haemophilus influenzae, Klebsiella pneumoniae*, group B Streptococcus [GBS], Ureaplasmas, *Mycomplasma hominis*, and *Neisseria gonorrhoeae*) have been identified using these techniques; in many cases, cultures reveal polymicrobial infection.[12–19]

More than 2 dozen randomized, controlled trials of adjunctive antibiotic therapy during conservative management of preterm PROM have been performed over the past 3 decades. These studies have been marked by a broad variety of treatment regimens, and variations in practice regarding antenatal corticosteroid administration, tocolytic therapy, GBS prophylaxis, and elective delivery. In many cases, patients with PROM in the late preterm period have been included, but these patients have limited potential to benefit from conservative management because achieved latency is brief and is associated with increased chorioamnionitis, and because serious newborn morbidity is infrequent with delivery at these gestational ages. Because the causative organisms are generally unknown with preterm PROM occurs, the optimal antibiotic regimen is unknown. Most studies have involved broad-spectrum antibiotic therapy given either intravenously or as a combination of intravenous and oral therapy.

Over the past 2 decades, several structured reviews of the published clinical trials have been performed, and a series of Cochrane Systematic reviews have been undertaken to address the utility of antibiotic treatment in this setting, and each has demonstrated some benefit from treatment.[20–22] The most recent review, updated by Kenyon and co-workers in the Cochrane Database of Systematic Reviews (2010), found that antibiotic treatment reduces the risk of chorioamnionitis (relative risk [RR], 0.66; 95% confidence interval [CI], 0.46–0.96) without significantly increasing other maternal morbidities.[22] Treatment reduces delivery within 48 hours of randomization (RR, 0.71; 95% CI, 0.58–0.87) and within 7 days (RR, 0.79; 95% CI, 0.71–0.89) of randomization. Moreover, such antibiotic treatment reduces neonatal infections (RR, 0.67; 95% CI, 0.52–0.85), major cerebral abnormalities (RR, 0.81; 95% CI, 0.68–0.98), and neonatal intensive care unit days (−5.05; 95% CI, −9.77 to −0.33) without decreasing or increasing the risk of necrotizing enterocolitis (RR, 1.09; 95% CI, 0.65–1.83) or respiratory distress syndrome (RR, 0.95; 95% CI, 0.83–1.09). However, this analysis included the broad range of treatments, including those utilizing narrow spectrum antibiotics, oral therapy alone, and those that included patients with PROM near term.

For the purposes of the article, further analysis was performed using a subgroup of available studies regarding this issue. Only prospected, controlled trials published in full manuscript form were included. Further, the analysis was restricted to studies that compared antibiotic treatment with a control or placebo group, recruited women at 34 weeks gestation or less, and initiated therapy with intravenous treatment, leaving 7 such studies for evaluation.[23–29] The goal of restricting the analysis in this way was to evaluate aggressive, broad-spectrum treatment given to those most likely to benefit and who would typically be managed conservatively after PROM. The analysis would have been restricted to women presenting before 32 weeks gestation, but only 2

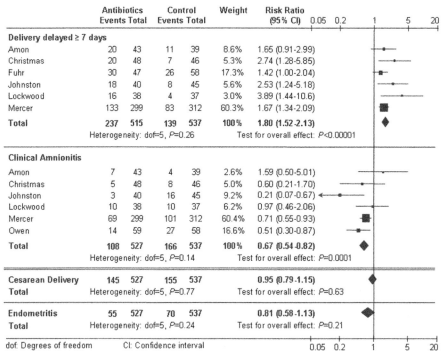

	Antibiotics		Control		Weight	Risk Ratio					
	Events	Total	Events	Total		(95% CI)	0.05	0.2	1	5	20
Delivery delayed ≥ 7 days											
Amon	20	43	11	39	8.6%	1.65 (0.91-2.99)					
Christmas	20	48	7	46	5.3%	2.74 (1.28-5.85)					
Fuhr	30	47	26	58	17.3%	1.42 (1.00-2.04)					
Johnston	18	40	8	45	5.6%	2.53 (1.24-5.18)					
Lockwood	16	38	4	37	3.0%	3.89 (1.44-10.6)					
Mercer	133	299	83	312	60.3%	1.67 (1.34-2.09)					
Total	**237**	**515**	**139**	**537**	**100%**	**1.80 (1.52-2.13)**					
Heterogeneity: dof=5, P=0.26					Test for overall effect: P<0.00001						
Clinical Amnionitis											
Amon	7	43	4	39	2.6%	1.59 (0.50-5.01)					
Christmas	5	48	8	46	5.0%	0.60 (0.21-1.70)					
Johnston	3	40	16	45	9.2%	0.21 (0.07-0.67)					
Lockwood	10	38	10	37	6.2%	0.97 (0.46-2.06)					
Mercer	69	299	101	312	60.4%	0.71 (0.55-0.93)					
Owen	14	59	27	58	16.6%	0.51 (0.30-0.87)					
Total	**108**	**527**	**166**	**537**	**100%**	**0.67 (0.54-0.82)**					
Heterogeneity: dof=5, P=0.14					Test for overall effect: P=0.0001						
Cesarean Delivery	145	527	155	537		0.95 (0.79-1.15)					
Total	Heterogeneity: dof=5, P=0.77					Test for overall effect: P=0.63					
Endometritis	55	527	70	537		0.81 (0.58-1.13)					
Total	Heterogeneity: dof=5, P=0.24					Test for overall effect: P=0.21					

dof: Degrees of freedom   CI: Confidence interval   0.05 0.2   1   5   20

Fig. 1. Meta-analysis of pregnancy outcomes associated with adjunctive antibiotic treatment versus control or placebo during conservative management of preterm premature rupture of the membranes at or before 34 weeks' gestation. (*Data from* figures generated by Review Manager. Version 5.0. Copenhagen: The Nordic Cochrane Centre, The Cochrane Collaboration, 2008.)

studies met this criterion.[23,24] Statistical analyses were performed using Review Manager (RevMan) Version 5.0. (Copenhagen, The Nordic Cochrane Centre, The Cochrane Collaboration, 2008). Mantel–Haenszel chi-square analyses, using a fixed-effects model, were performed. Data are presented as summary RRs (95% CI). Heterogeneity was evaluated using the Q statistic, with P-values for the summary RRs.

The results of this analysis are presented in **Figs. 1** and **2**. To conserve space, only the summary statistics are presented for outcomes in which statistical significance was not reached. In summary, broad-spectrum adjunctive antibiotic treatment with initial parenteral therapy during conservative management of PROM at or before 34 weeks gestation results in improved latency (delivery ≥7 days, 46.0% vs 25.9%) and less frequent amnionitis (20.5% vs 31.3%) without increasing the risks of cesarean delivery (27.5% vs 28.5%) or the rate of postpartum endometritis (10.5% vs 13.0%; Fig. 1). Such treatment results in less frequent newborn sepsis (10.9% vs 16.8%) as well as less frequent gestational age-dependent morbidities, including respiratory distress syndrome (37.9% vs 46.2%) and intraventricular hemorrhage (12.9% vs 17.8%; Fig. 2). Aggressive, broad-spectrum, adjunctive antibiotic treatment is not associated with altered rates of necrotizing enterocolitis (8.2% vs 6.9%), stillbirth (0.9% vs 2.7%), or survival to discharge (93.7% vs 92.4%). Despite the cohort being

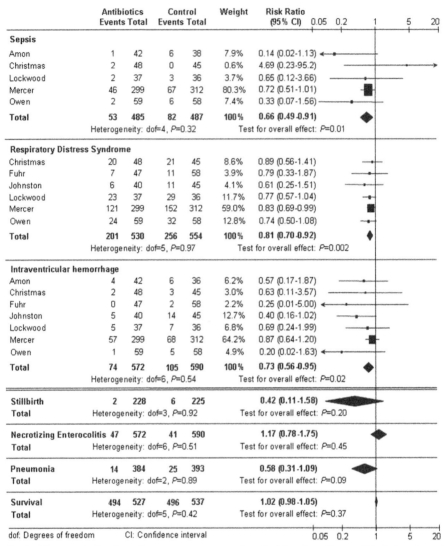

Fig. 2. Meta-analysis of newborn outcomes associated with adjunctive antibiotic treatment versus control or placebo during conservative management of preterm PROM at or before 34 weeks' gestation. (*Data from* figures generated by Review Manager. Version 5.0. Copenhagen: The Nordic Cochrane Centre, The Cochrane Collaboration, 2008.)

restricted to pregnancies at or before 34 weeks gestation, the overall rate of stillbirth was infrequent (1.8%), and survival to discharge was common (93%).

Several individual studies provide added insights regarding this practice. In a placebo-controlled trial of oral erythromycin therapy published in 1992, we found treatment to prolong pregnancy, but not reduce maternal or newborn infections, or gestational age-dependent morbidities.[30] Antibiotic treatment significantly prolonged pregnancy among women destined to develop clinical chorioamnionitis. By comparison, a larger, placebo-controlled study of oral erythromycin therapy for preterm

PROM, the ORACLE I trial, found reductions in newborn need for surfactant with erythromycin treatment alone, but no reductions in other morbidities, and no improvement in latency beyond 48 hours.[31] Alternatively, a trial conducted by the Eunice Kennedy Shriver National Institutes of Child Health and Human Development Maternal Fetal Medicine Units Research Network (NICHD-MFMU), found improved latency at each day between 2 days and 3 weeks after randomization, despite antibiotics being discontinued at 7 days for those who remained undelivered.[23] This suggests that broad-spectrum treatment not only suppressed subclinical infection during treatment, but actually successfully treated it.

The 2 largest trials published regarding antibiotic therapy after PROM deserve specific attention. The first was undertaken by the NICHD-MFMU Network and was adequately powered to evaluate the impact of antibiotic treatment on newborn morbidities in addition to latency.[23] In this randomized, double-blind, placebo-controlled trial participants with preterm PROM between 24^0 and 32^0 weeks gestation were assigned to receive intravenous ampicillin and erythromycin for 48 hours, followed by oral amoxicillin and erythromycin for up to 5 days or matching placebo if undelivered. Those with a positive GBS culture received ampicillin for 7 days, and were treated again in labor. Antenatal corticosteroids were not administered. Overall, subjects assigned to antibiotic treatment had less frequent newborn composite morbidity (44.1% vs 52.9%; $P = .04$), respiratory distress (40.5% vs 48.7%; $P = .04$), and stage 2 or 3 necrotizing enterocolitis (2.3% vs 5.8%; $P = .03$), and chronic lung disease (bronchopulmonary dysplasia, 13.0% vs 20.5%; $P = .01$) in addition to less frequent amnionitis (23.0% vs 32.5%; $P = .01$). Regarding newborn infectious outcomes, broad-spectrum antibiotic treatment reduced the frequencies of neonatal sepsis (8.4% vs 15.6%; $P = .01$) and pneumonia (2.9% vs 7.0%; $P = .04$) among those who were not GBS carriers. Of note, GBS carriers in the placebo group received 1 week of ampicillin as well as intrapartum therapy, so the benefit of broad-spectrum treatment would be expected to be less apparent in this subgroup and did not attain significance. Overall, this study found that practice of initiating broad-spectrum treatment, and giving intrapartum prophylaxis to identified GBS carriers during conservative management of preterm PROM at 32^0 weeks gestation or less, resulted in pregnancy prolongation, and reduced infectious and gestational age-dependent morbidities without increasing perinatal complications.

The second large study, the ORACLE I trial, included 4826 women with PROM before 37 weeks who were randomized to 10 days of oral erythromycin (n = 1197), amoxicillin-clavulanic acid (n = 1212), both (n = 1192), or a matching placebo regimen (n = 1225).[31] This study was also adequately powered to evaluate the impact of antibiotic treatments on newborn outcomes, but women were conservatively managed with PROM occurring up to 36^6 weeks gestation. In summary, this group found that oral erythromycin treatment alone was associated with only brief pregnancy prolongation, as noted (34.8% vs 40.7% delivered at 48 hours; $P = .004$) but not within 7 days (60.9% vs 63.3%; $P = -.23$). Oral erythromycin treatment reduced the need for supplemental oxygen (31.1% vs 35.6%; $P = .02$) and resulted in less frequent positive blood cultures (5.7% vs 8.2%; $P = .02$). Oral amoxicillin-clavulanic acid treatment alone prolonged pregnancy (57.7% vs 63.3% delivered within 7 days; $P = .005$) and reduced the need for supplemental oxygen (30.1% vs 35.6%; $P = .05$). However, this study found oral amoxicillin-clavulanic acid treatment alone to increase the risk of necrotizing enterocolitis (1.9% vs 0.5%; $P = .001$). This finding is at odds with the NICHD-MFMU study, which found antibiotics to prevent stage 2 to 3 necrotizing enterocolitis in the overall cohort. Further, the published meta-analyses reveal no consistent pattern of increased risk for necrotizing enterocolitis with antibiotic treatments. Regardless, based on this study and the availability of other treatments, it would be prudent to avoid oral amoxicillin clavulanic acid in this setting. The ORACLE I trial is the only large study of conservatively managed PROM that obtained long-term infant follow-up.[32] Seven-year follow-up of these infants using a structured parental questionnaire revealed no evident differences between antibiotic and control groups regarding medical conditions, behavioral difficulties, or functional impairment.

Two subsequent studies have attempted to determine whether the duration of adjunctive antibiotic therapy during conservative management of preterm PROM could be shortened, but are of inadequate size and power to evaluate infant outcomes adequately.[33,34]

There are a number of factors that may impact our interpretation of the published literature. Inclusion of women with PROM near term or before fetal viability confounds the potential to identify significant infant benefit from antibiotic treatment. Brief pregnancy prolongation at 20 to 22 weeks gestation could result in live-birth of a child at high risk for gestational age-dependent morbidities with periviable birth, whereas brief pregnancy prolongation at 34 to 36 weeks gestation is unlikely to dramatically reduce gestational age-dependent complications. From the ORACLE I trial, it seems that oral therapy alone is inadequate in the setting of preterm PROM. But a number of the published studies did not provide parenteral therapy, but are included in published meta-analyses of antibiotic treatment: Not all antibiotic regimens are the same. Several of the diagnoses evaluated in the published literature could be affected by the administration of antibiotics. Clinical chorioamnionitis may be less frequently diagnosed after antibiotic treatment if therapy reduces the number of women with a fever. Regarding the neonate, a diagnosis of confirmed sepsis generally requires a positive blood culture, and persistent neonatal blood antibiotic levels after maternal administration may lead to negative neonatal cultures (a microbiologic artifact) and prevent the diagnosis of "confirmed" or "proven" sepsis. Alternatively, if antibiotic treatment prevents the diagnosis of chorioamnionitis or early neonatal infection, we would anticipate less frequent therapy for these with an increase in the diagnosis of delayed-onset morbidities. These have not been reported with antibiotic treatment in this setting.

Based on these findings, optimal adjunctive antibiotic treatment of preterm PROM should be restricted to pregnancies where pregnancy prolongation is likely to result in a reduction of newborn gestational age-dependent morbidities, and where the risk of neonatal death is greater than the 1% to 2% risk of stillbirth with conservative management. Antibiotic treatment should generally include initial aggressive, broad-spectrum intravenous therapy. In the absence of data demonstrating equivalency of 3- and 7-day antibiotic regimens in terms of reducing newborn complications and not just latency, regimens that have demonstrated reductions in both newborn infectious and gestational age-dependent morbidity with significant pregnancy prolongation are recommended. Our current practice is to give intravenous ampicillin and erythromycin for 48 hours, followed by an oral regimen of amoxicillin and erythromycin for an additional 5 days if delivery does not occur. GBS carriers and those delivering before cultures become available require intrapartum prophylaxis with penicillin (or an appropriate alternative for penicillin-allergic women) unless broader spectrum therapy for chorioamnionitis is required.

ANTIBIOTICS FOR PRETERM LABOR

Given the promising findings regarding the beneficial effects of antibiotic treatment during conservative management of preterm PROM, one would hope that antibiotic treatment in the setting of preterm labor would offer similar benefits. A significant fraction of women presenting with preterm labor have positive amniotic fluid cultures. As is the case with preterm PROM, a broad range of organisms have been identified from amniocentesis specimens by culture and polymerase chain reaction; bacterial colonization is associated with relatively brief latency to delivery after presentation, and chorioamnionitis is a frequent finding after delivery owing to preterm labor.[35–37]

Several early studies revealed promising results regarding the potential for a benefit from adjunctive antibiotic treatment for preterm labor. McGregor and colleagues,[36] in 1986, randomized participants to oral erythromycin or a matching placebo and found significant pregnancy prolongation with antibiotic treatment (32.5 vs 22.4 days; P = .027); these women were more likely to deliver at term.[38] However, these investigators were unable to replicate these findings in a subsequent study of intravenous clindamycin therapy,[39] and neither study demonstrated reductions in newborn morbidities. In a study of ampicillin or erythromycin versus placebo, Morales and associates[40] found improved latency with antibiotic treatment (31.7 and 28.5 vs 16.6 days; $P<.01$ and $P<.05$, respectively). Winkler and co-investigators,[41] in a study of oral erythromycin versus placebo, found improved latency among women with cultures positive for *Ureaplasma urealyticum* (43 vs 20 days; $P<.05$), but no benefit was seen in culture-negative women. Norman and co-investigators,[42] in 1994, found intravenous ampicillin and oral metronidazole to prolong pregnancy (15 vs 2.5 days; $P<.04$) and also to lead to less frequent necrotizing enterocolitis (0% vs 13.9%; P = .02). One study found more advanced gestational age at delivery (36.6 vs 33.8 weeks; $P<.05$), and suggested reductions in neonatal infectious morbidity, intrauterine growth restriction, histologic chorioamnionitis, and postpartum endometritis with ampicillin treatment (1 g orally 3 times daily for 7 days).[43] Most impressively, in a randomized controlled study by Svare and colleagues in 1997,[44] in which 112 patients with idiopathic preterm labor were assigned to 24 hours of intravenous followed by 7 days of oral therapy with ampicillin and metronidazole or placebo, antibiotic treatment was associated with prolonged latency (47.5 vs 27 days; $P<.05$), less frequent preterm birth (42% vs 65%; $P<.05$), and fewer neonatal intensive care unit admissions (40% vs 63%; $P<.05$), but no reductions in perinatal morbidities were identified. Alternatively, studies by Newton and co-workers[45,46] in 1989 and 1991, McCaul (1992),[47] Romero (1993),[48] and Cox (1996)[49] and their co-workers found no benefits regarding pregnancy prolongation or reduction in newborn morbidities with antibiotic treatment given adjunctively during the acute management of preterm labor.

These prior studies are overshadowed by the ORACLE II trial in which women with preterm labor with intact membranes before 36 weeks gestation were randomly assigned to oral amoxicillin-clavulanic acid, erythromycin, both, or placebo.[50] In this large, adequately powered study of 6295 subjects, no improvements in latency or newborn infectious or gestational age-dependent morbidities were identified with antibiotic treatment given either individually or in combination. Importantly these investigators conducted a 7-year follow-up study of infants delivered from the study using a structured questionnaire.[51] A surprising finding was that infants exposed to antibiotic treatment in utero were had more frequent functional impairment and cerebral palsy. This finding is mitigated by the lack of objective examinations, and the lack of a similar finding in the ORACLE I study of preterm PROM in which infants would be expected to have a higher incidence of neurologic complications but did not.

Several meta-analyses have been performed to assess the efficacy of adjunctive antibiotic therapy to prolong pregnancy for the purpose of reducing gestational age dependent and infectious newborn morbidities. King and associates,[52] in a Cochrane review included 11 trials and found no improvements in delivery within 48 hours (RR,

1.04; 95% CI, 0.89–1.23), 7 days (RR, 0.98; 95% CI, 0.87–1.10), preterm birth (RR, 0.99; 95% CI, 0.92–1.05), or major newborn morbidities, including respiratory distress syndrome (RR, 0.99; 95% CI, 0.84–1.16), intraventricular hemorrhage (RR, 0.76; 95% CI, 0.66–1.51), sepsis (RR, 0.86; 95% CI, 0.64–1.16), necrotizing enterocolitis (RR, 1.06; 95% CI, 0.64–1.73), or perinatal mortality (RR, 1.22; 95% CI, 0.88–1.70). Similarly, Hutzal and colleagues[53] found little evidence of benefit from administration of adjunctive antibiotics in the treatment of preterm labor at or before 34 weeks' gestation.

The literature regarding adjunctive antibiotic treatment for preterm labor is somewhat limited by the fact that intrauterine uterine infection is less frequently present in this scenario than in the setting of PROM, and that many such women proceed to term in the absence of specific treatment with antibiotics or tocolytic agents. Given this, antibiotic administration to all women with idiopathic preterm labor would result in treatment of many who could not potentially benefit. The availability of technologies to identify those who might truly benefit from antibiotic treatment could potentially change this approach. For example, symptomatic women with preterm contractions and a short cervical length or a positive fetal fibronectin screen remote from term are at increased risk for delivery within a short period of time.[54–57] These women might potentially benefit from antibiotic treatment; however, this hypothesis has not been studied. The potential for risks from antibiotic treatment should also be considered. Prenatal exposure of the fetus to maternal antibiotics is associated with an increased risk of antibiotic-resistant sepsis.[58–60]

Aggressive intravenous and oral adjunctive antibiotic therapy during acute management of idiopathic preterm labor is not associated with consistent improvement in latency or improvements in newborn outcomes. Given this, and the potential for risks from intrauterine antibiotic exposure in this setting, antibiotic treatment for pregnancy prolongation and reduction of infant morbidity is not recommended. Antibiotic treatment of preterm labor should be reserved for women with clear indications, such as known acute infections amenable to antibiotic therapy, intrapartum GBS prophylaxis, and chorioamnionitis.

SUMMARY

A significant fraction of preterm birth results from subclinical intrauterine infection. It is presumed that ascending bacterial colonization of the decidua results and either uterine contractions or membrane weakening that results in the clinical presentation of preterm labor or PROM. Those with overt infection require delivery. However, it is plausible that adjunctive antibiotic treatment during therapy for preterm labor and PROM remote from term could result in pregnancy prolongation and reductions in gestational age-dependent and infectious newborn morbidities. Data support adjunctive antibiotic treatment during conservative management of PROM remote from term. Such treatment should include broad-spectrum agents, typically intravenous therapy initially, and continue for up to 7 days if undelivered. Such treatment should be reserved for women presenting remote from term where significant improvement in neonatal outcomes can be anticipated with conservative management. Alternatively, current evidence suggests that antibiotic treatment in the setting of preterm labor with intact membranes does not consistently prolong pregnancy or improve newborn outcomes. Given this, and the concerning findings from the ORACLE II trial of antibiotics for preterm labor, this treatment should not be offered in the setting of preterm labor with intact membranes. Although one could speculate that women with preterm labor and with either a short cervical length for a positive fetal fibronectin screen might benefit from antibiotic therapy, no well-designed, randomized, controlled trials addressing this issue have been completed. Therefore, antibiotic therapy for women in preterm labor should be reserved for usual clinical indications, including suspected bacterial infections, GBS prophylaxis, and chorioamnionitis.

REFERENCES

1. Goldenberg RL, Culhane JF, Iams JD, et al. Epidemiology and causes of preterm birth. Lancet 2008;371:75–84.
2. Hillier SL, Martius J, Krohn M, et al. A case-control study of chorioamnionitis infection and histologic chorioamnionitis in prematurity. N Engl J Med 1988;319:972–8.
3. Hillier SL, Witkin SS, Krohn MA, et al. The relationship of amniotic fluid cytokines and preterm delivery, amniotic fluid infection, histologic chorioamnionitis, and chorioamnion infection. Obstet Gynecol 1993;81:941–8.
4. Gibbs RS, Romero R, Hillier SL, et al. A review of premature birth and subclinical infection. Am J Obstet Gynecol 1991;166:1515–28.
5. Minkoff H. Prematurity: infection as an etiologic factor. Obstet Gynecol 1993;62: 137–44.
6. McDonald HM, Brocklehurst P, Gordon A. Antibiotics for treating bacterial vaginosis in pregnancy. Cochrane Database Syst Rev 2007;1:CD00262.
7. Romero R, Oyarzun E, Mazor M, et al. Meta-Analysis of the relationship between asymptomatic bacteriuria and preterm delivery/low birth weight. Obstet Gynecol 1989;73:576–82.
8. Carey BV, Eschenbach DA, Nugent RP, et al; the Vaginal Infections and Prematurity Study Group. A randomized placebo-controlled trial of erythromycin for the treatment of Ureaplasma urealyticum to prevent premature delivery. Am J Obstet Gynecol 1991;164:734–42.
9. Klebanoff MA, Carey JC, Hauth JC, et al; National Institute of Child Health and Human Development Network of Maternal-Fetal Medicine Units. Failure of metronidazole to prevent preterm delivery among pregnant women with asymptomatic Trichomonas vaginalis infection. N Engl J Med 2001;345:487–93.
10. Andrews WW, Goldenberg RL, Hauth JC, et al. Interconceptional antibiotics to prevent spontaneous preterm birth: a randomized clinical trial. Am J Obstet Gynecol 2006;194:617–23.
11. Andrews WW, Sibai BM, Thom EA, et al; National Institute of Child Health & Human Development Maternal-Fetal Medicine Units Network. Randomized clinical trial of metronidazole plus erythromycin to prevent spontaneous preterm delivery in fetal fibronectin-positive women. Obstet Gynecol 2003;101:847–55.
12. Broekhuizen FF, Gilman M. Hamilton PR. Amniocentesis for gram stain and culture in preterm premature rupture of the membranes. Obstet Gynecol 1985;66:316–21.
13. Cotton DB, Hill LM, Strassner HT, et al. The use of amniocentesis in preterm gestation with ruptured membranes. Obstet Gynecol 1984;63:38–43.
14. Zlatnik FJ, Cruickshank DP, Petzold CR, et al. Amniocentesis in the identification of inapparent infection in preterm patients with premature rupture of the membranes. J Reprod Med 1984;29:656–60.
15. Mercer B, Moretti M, Rogers R, et al. Antibiotic prophylaxis in preterm premature rupture of the membranes: A prospective randomized double-blind trial of 220 patients. Am J Obstet Gynecol 1992;166:794–802.
16. Romero R, Emamian M, Quintero R, et al. The value and limitations of the gram stain examination in the diagnosis of intra-amniotic infection. Am J Obstet Gynecol 1988; 159:114–9.

17. Wager GP, Hanley LS, Farb HF, et al. Evaluation of gas-liquid chromatography for the rapid diagnosis of amniotic fluid infection: a preliminary report. Am J Obstet Gynecol 1985;152:51–6.
18. Oh KJ, Lee KA, Sohn YK, et al. Intraamniotic infection with genital mycoplasmas exhibits a more intense inflammatory response than intraamniotic infection with other microorganisms in patients with preterm premature rupture of membranes. Am J Obstet Gynecol 2010;203:211.e1–8.
19. DiGiulio DB, Romero R, Kusanovic JP, et al. Prevalence and diversity of microbes in the amniotic fluid, the fetal inflammatory response, and pregnancy outcome in women with preterm pre-labor rupture of membranes. Am J Reprod Immunol 2010 1;64:38–57.
20. Mercer BM, Arheart K. Antimicrobial therapy in expectant management of preterm premature rupture of the membranes. Lancet 1995;346:1271–9.
21. Egarter C, Leitich H, Karas H, et al. Antibiotic treatment in preterm premature rupture of membranes and neonatal morbidity: a metaanalysis. Am J Obstet Gynecol 1996; 174:589–97.
22. Kenyon S, Boulvain M, Neilson JP. Antibiotics for preterm rupture of membranes. Cochrane Database Syst Rev 2010;8:CD001058.
23. Mercer B, Miodovnik M, Thurnau G, et al; the NICHD-MFMU Network. Antibiotic therapy for reduction of infant morbidity after preterm premature rupture of the membranes: a randomized controlled trial. JAMA 1997;278:989–95.
24. Lockwood CJ, Costigan K, Ghidini A, et al. Double-blind placebo-controlled trial of piperacillin prophylaxis in preterm membrane rupture. Am J Obstet Gynecol 1993; 169:970–6.
25. Amon E, Lewis SV, Sibai BM, et al. Ampicillin prophylaxis in preterm premature rupture of the membranes: a prospective randomized study. Am J Obstet Gynecol 1988;159:539–43.
26. Johnston MM, Sanchez-Ramos L, Vaughn AJ, et al. Antibiotic therapy in preterm premature rupture of the membranes: a randomized prospective double-blind trial. Am J Obstet Gynecol 1990;163:743–7.
27. Christmas JT, Cox SM, Andrews W, et al. Expectant management of preterm ruptured membranes: Effects of antimicrobial therapy. Obstet Gynecol 1992;80: 759–62.
28. Owen J, Groome LJ, Hauth JC. Randomized trial of prophylactic antibiotic therapy after preterm amnion rupture. Am J Obstet Gynecol 1993;169:976–81.
29. Fuhr N, Becker C, van Baalen A, et al. Antibiotic therapy for preterm premature rupture of membranes: results of a multicenter study. J Perinat Med 2006;34:203–6.
30. Mercer BM, Moretti ML, Prevost RR, et al. Erythromycin therapy in preterm premature rupture of the membranes: a prospective, randomized trial of 220 patients. Am J Obstet Gynecol 1992;166:794–802.
31. Kenyon SL, Taylor DJ, Tarnow-Mordi W; Oracle Collaborative Group. Broad spectrum antibiotics for preterm, prelabor rupture of fetal membranes: the ORACLE I Randomized trial. Lancet 2001;357:979–88.
32. Kenyon S, Pike K, Jones DR, et al. Childhood outcomes after prescription of antibiotics to pregnant women with preterm rupture of the membranes: 7-year follow-up of the ORACLE I trial. Lancet 2008;372:1310–8.
33. Lewis DF, Adair CD, Robichaux AG, et al. Antibiotic therapy in preterm premature rupture of membranes: are seven days necessary? A preliminary, randomized clinical trial. Am J Obstet Gynecol 2003;188:1413–6.
34. Segel SY, Miles AM, Clothier B, et al. Duration of antibiotic therapy after preterm premature rupture of fetal membranes. Am J Obstet Gynecol 2003;189:799–802.

35. Skoll MA, Moretti ML, Sibai BM. The incidence of positive amniotic fluid cultures in patients preterm labor with intact membranes. Am J Obstet Gynecol 1989;161: 813–6.

36. Romero R, Sirtori M, Oyarzun E, et al. Infection and labor. V. Prevalence, microbiology, and clinical significance of intraamniotic infection in women with preterm labor and intact membranes. Am J Obstet Gynecol 1989;161:817–24.

37. DiGiulio DB, Romero R, Amogan HP, et al. Microbial prevalence, diversity and abundance in amniotic fluid during preterm labor: a molecular and culture-based investigation. PLoS One 2008;3:e3056.

38. McGregor JA, French JI, Reller LB, et al. Adjunctive erythromycin treatment for idiopathic preterm labor: results of a randomized, double-blinded placebo-controlled trial. Am J Obstet Gynecol 1986;154:98–103.

39. McGregor JA, French JI, Seo K. Adjunctive clindamycin therapy for preterm labor results of a double-blind, placebo-controlled trial. Am J Obstet Gynecol 1991;165: 867–75.

40. Morales WJ, Angel JD, O'Brien WF, et al. A randomized study of antibiotic therapy in idiopathic preterm labor. Obstet Gynecol 1988;72:829–33.

41. Winkler M, Baumann L, Ruchhäberle KE, et al. Erythromycin therapy for subclinical intrauterine infections in threatened preterm delivery: a preliminary report. J Perinatal Med 1988;16:253–6.

42. Norman K, Pattison RC, de Souza J, et al. Ampicillin and metronidazole treatment in preterm labour: a multicentre, randomised controlled trial. Br J Obstet Gynecol 1994;101:404–8.

43. Nadisauskiene R, Bergstrom S, Kilda A. Ampicillin in the treatment of preterm labor: a randomised, placebo-controlled study. Gynecol Obstet Invest 1996;41:89–92.

44. Svare J, Langhoff-Roos J, Anderson LF, et al. Ampicillin-metronidazole treatment in idiopathic preterm labour: a randomised controlled muticentre trial. Br J Obstet Gynecol 1997;104:892–7.

45. Newton ER, Dinsmoor MJ, Gibbs RS. A randomized, blinded, placebo-controlled trial of antibiotics in idiopathic preterm labor. Obstet Gynecol 1989;74:562–6.

46. Newton ER, Shields L, Ridgway LE III, et al. Combination antibiotics and indomethacin in idiopathic preterm labor: a randomized double-blind clinical trial. Am J Obstet Gynecol 1991;165:1753–9.

47. McCaul JF, Perry KG, Moore JL, et al. Adjunctive antibiotic treatment of women with preterm rupture of membranes or preterm labor. Int J Gynaecol Obstet 1992;38:19–24.

48. Romero R, Sibai BM, Caritis S, et al. Antibiotic treatment of preterm labor with intact membranes: a multicenter, randomized, double-blinding, placebo-controlled trial. Am J Obstet Gynecol 1993;169:764–74.

49. Cox SM, Bohman VR, Sherman ML, et al. Randomized investigation of antimicrobials for the prevention of preterm birth. Am J Obstet Gynecol 1996;174:206–10.

50. Kenyon SL, Taylor DJ, Tarnow-Mordi W; ORACLE Collaborative Group. Broad-spectrum antibiotics for spontaneous preterm labour: the ORACLE II randomised trial. ORACLE Collaborative Group. Lancet 2001;357:989–94.

51. Kenyon S, Pike K, Jones DR, et al. Childhood outcomes after prescription of antibiotics to pregnant women with spontaneous preterm labour: 7-year follow-up of the ORACLE II trial. Lancet 2008;372:1319–27.

52. King J, Flenady V. Prophylactic antibiotics for inhibiting preterm labour with intact membranes. Cochrane Database Syst Rev 2002;4:CD000246.

53. Hutzal CE, Boyle EM, Kenyon SL, et al. Use of antibiotics for the treatment of preterm parturition and prevention of neonatal morbidity: a metaanalysis. Am J Obstet Gynecol 2008;199:620, e1–8.

54. Tsoi E, Akmal S, Rane S, et al. Ultrasound assessment of cervical length in threatened preterm labor. Ultrasound Obstet Gynecol 2003;21:552–5.

55. Fuchs I, Tsoi E, Henrich W, et al. Sonographic measurement of cervical length in twin pregnancies in threatened preterm labor. Ultrasound Obstet Gynecol 2004;23:42–5.

56. Tsoi E, Akmal S, Geerts L, et al. Sonographic measurement of cervical length and fetal fibronectin testing in threatened preterm labor. Ultrasound Obstet Gynecol 2006;27: 368–72.

57. Schmitz T, Maillard F, Bessard-Bacquaert S, et al. Selective use of fetal fibronectin detection after cervical length measurement to predict spontaneous preterm delivery in women with preterm labor. Am J Obstet Gynecol 2006;194:138–43.

58. Mercer BM, Carr TL, Beazley DD, et al. Antibiotic use in pregnancy and drug-resistant infant sepsis. Am J Obstet Gynecol 1999;181:816–21.

59. Terrone DA, Rinehart BK, Einstein MH, et al. Neonatal sepsis and death caused by resistant Escherichia coli; Possible consequences of extended maternal ampicillin administration. Am J Obstet Gynecol 1999;180:1345–8.

60. Bizzarro MJ, Dembry L, Baltimore RS, et al. Changing patterns in neonatal Escherichia coli sepsis and ampicillin resistance in the era of intrapartum antibiotic prophylaxis. Pediatrics 2008;121:689–96.

Tocolytic Therapy for Acute Preterm Labor

Adi Abramovici, MD*, Jessica Cantu, MD, Sheri M. Jenkins, MD

KEYWORDS

- Preterm labor • Tocolytic therapy • Magnesium sulfate
- Beta-mimetics • Calcium channel blockers
- Prostaglandin inhibitors • Oxytocin receptor antagonist

Preterm birth is the leading cause of perinatal morbidity and mortality and leads to significant health care costs annually. Despite numerous advances in the care of obstetrical patients, the incidence of preterm birth in the United States is at an all-time high and may be on the rise given current trends of advancing maternal age, maternal medical conditions, assisted reproductive technology, and multiple gestations.[1] Neonatal morbidity is strongly associated with gestational age at birth with adverse neonatal outcomes occurring in 77% of those born at 24 to 27 weeks' gestation compared with only 2% born at or beyond 34 weeks.[2] Therefore, prevention of preterm birth and its associated neonatal morbidity and mortality are major worldwide concerns and a significant focus for obstetrical research.

Certain maternal factors have been identified that increase the risk of preterm birth. African-American women have consistently higher rates of preterm birth ranging from 16% to 18% compared with 5% to 9% of Caucasian women.[3] Also, women with a prior history of preterm birth have a 2.5-fold increased risk of preterm delivery in a subsequent pregnancy,[4] although this risk may be reduced with progesterone supplementation.[5,6] Additional risk factors include low socioeconomic status, poor nutritional status, maternal medical conditions, extremes of maternal age, smoking, and history of cervical conization.

Preterm labor is thought to be a multifactorial process with an underlying infection as the initiating factor in at least 25% to 40% of preterm births.[3] Microorganisms within the upper genital tract cause activation of the immune response with production of inflammatory cytokines and prostaglandins that result in uterine contractions and weakening of the amniotic membranes. Despite this association between infection and preterm delivery, antibiotics have not been shown to decrease the risk for preterm birth.[7] Tocolytics have also not been shown to decrease the risk for

The authors have nothing to disclose.
Division of Maternal-Fetal Medicine, University of Alabama, Birmingham, 619 19th Street South 176F 10270C, Birmingham, AL 35249-7333, USA
* Corresponding author.
E-mail address: adi.abramovici@obgyn.uab.edu

preterm birth, but they have been shown to temporarily inhibit uterine contractions. In a systematic review including 18 randomized, controlled trials comparing a tocolytic versus placebo or no treatment for preterm labor, tocolysis decreased the risk of delivery within 48 hours and 7 days, but did not prevent preterm birth before 37 weeks.[8]

Given the short-term delay in delivery with tocolysis, the primary goal of tocolytic therapy is to allow administration of glucocorticoids to reduce the risk of the prematurity-related complications of respiratory distress syndrome, necrotizing enterocolitis, and intraventricular hemorrhage. In addition, a second goal of tocolytics is to allow for maternal transport to a facility capable of providing more advanced neonatal care. Tocolysis may be discontinued when these goals are met or when the maternal or fetal risk of pregnancy continuation or drug exposure outweighs the morbidity associated with preterm birth, generally around 34 weeks' gestation.[9] Contraindications to tocolysis include evidence of intra-amniotic infection, intrauterine fetal demise, lethal fetal anomalies, severe fetal growth restriction, preeclampsia, or nonreassuring fetal status. In this article, we review the various tocolytics used for preterm labor and examine their mechanisms of action, efficacy, dosing, and side effects.

MAGNESIUM SULFATE

Magnesium sulfate is the most commonly used tocolytic agent in the United States.[10] It was first evaluated for tocolysis in the 1970s.[11] Although the mechanism of action is not completely understood, it is thought to be related to its antagonistic action with calcium. A predominant portion (99%) of magnesium is intracellular, localized to bones, myocytes, nuclei, microsomes, and mitochondria. Of the 1% that is extracellular, 62% circulates ionized in the maternal serum.[12,13] Magnesium functions at the extracellular and intracellular levels, decreasing the availability of calcium by blocking membrane and intracellular calcium channels, which decreases myometrial contractility.[14,15]

Magnesium sulfate has failed to show benefit or superior efficacy to other tocolytics in multiple systematic reviews, yet it is still commonly used today. In a systematic review of 4 randomized trials evaluating the efficacy of magnesium sulfate compared with placebo or no therapy for preterm labor, there was no reduction in the frequency of delivery within 48 hours, 7 days, or before 37 weeks gestation. There was also not a reduction in the outcome of newborn birth weight of less than 2500 grams. In addition, no single study was able to show an improvement in the more common newborn morbidities of respiratory distress, intraventricular hemorrhage, necrotizing enterocolitis, and sepsis.[16] Comparison of magnesium sulfate with other tocolytic regimens does not show magnesium to be more efficacious than other tocolytics. In this same systematic review, magnesium sulfate was compared with beta-mimetics, calcium channel blockers, and cyclooxygenase (COX) inhibitors in 15 studies. Magnesium sulfate did not show improved length of gestation or neonatal benefit compared with the other tocolytics.

Standard administration doses for magnesium include a 4- to 6-g loading dose over 20 to 30 minutes followed by a continuous infusion of 2 g/h. Titration may be necessary depending on contraction frequency and tolerance of drug. It is contraindicated in women with myasthenia gravis and should be used in caution in the setting of renal insufficiency because it is excreted by the kidneys. Impaired renal function may quickly lead to toxicity at normal doses. In patients with renal insufficiency (serum creatinine >1.0 mg/dL), a loading dose is acceptable but the maintenance dose should be held or kept at 1 g/h.[17]

Maternal side effects, which range from mild to severe, are seen in up to 60% of exposed women and include flushing, nausea, blurry vision, headache, lethargy, hypotension, and pulmonary edema.[18,19] Magnesium toxicity is related to serum concentration level. Loss of patellar reflexes may be the first clinical sign of toxicity followed by decreased urine output (<100 mL/4 h). Reflexes and urine output should be monitored closely during administration.[17] Although rare, respiratory depression and arrest can occur at levels above 10 to 12 mg/dL, so the medication should be stopped and serum level checked if there is clinical concern for toxicity.

Controversy around the effect of magnesium sulfate on the fetus and neonate has been cited in the literature. Magnesium has been shown to decrease fetal heart rate baseline and variability, but these do not have clinical significance.[20] Other studies have shown adverse neonatal effects from magnesium exposure. In a randomized, controlled trial by Lyell and colleages[19] comparing magnesium sulfate with nifedipine for tocolysis, infants exposed to magnesium had an increased rate of neonatal intensive care unit (NICU) admission and longer NICU stays. Other authors have suggested that magnesium sulfate slows gastrointestinal function and may lead to respiratory suppression.[21] Last, a Cochrane review of seven studies in 2002 found an increased risk for perinatal death with prenatal exposure to magnesium[22]; however, a more recent systematic review showed no increase in fetal or neonatal death before discharge for magnesium compared with any alternative tocolytic regimen or control group.[16]

Despite potential adverse neonatal effects, contrary evidence has suggested that prenatal exposure to magnesium may have a neuroprotective benefit. A randomized, controlled trial by Crowther and associates[23] evaluating the neuroprotective effect of magnesium given before preterm birth found an almost a 50% reduction in gross motor dysfunction (3.4% vs 6.6%) in the group treated with magnesium sulfate compared with placebo.[23] These findings were supported by Marret and co-workers,[24] who demonstrated a reduction in death or motor/cognitive dysfunction among the group receiving magnesium sulfate. In 2008, a randomized controlled trial by Rouse and coleageus[25] examined the role of magnesium sulfate for the prevention of cerebral palsy in 2241 patients. The study was conducted among women at gestational ages of 24 to 31 6/7 weeks who received a standard 6-g loading dose followed by a continuous infusion of 2g/h until the time of delivery. The study showed a 45% reduction in the overall rate of cerebral palsy (4.2% vs 7.3%) and in moderate or severe cerebral palsy (1.9% vs 3.5%) in the infants receiving magnesium.

Although it is widely used as a tocolytic agent, the literature does not support magnesium sulfate as being effective in withholding delivery for 48 hours, preventing preterm birth, or reducing the risk for neonatal morbidity. Given its association with the reduction in the rate of cerebral palsy, magnesium's best role seems to be as a neuroprotective agent for the fetus.

BETA-MIMETICS

The role of beta-mimetics for tocolysis has been explored since the 1970s.[26–28] Medications belonging to this class include terbutaline (Brethine), ritodrine (Yutopar), salbutamol, and hexoprenaline. Ritodrine is the only Food and Drug Administration-approved tocolytic medication, but it is no longer available in the United States.[17] Although beta-mimetics were initially commonly used, they have fallen out of favor secondary to their maternal and fetal side effects and a recent warning released in February 2011 by the US Food and Drug Administration. The US Food and Drug Administration placed a boxed warning on the drug's label stating that the medication should not be used for prolonged tocolysis (>48–72 hours) because of the potential for serious maternal cardiac toxicity and death.[29]

Beta-mimetics function as beta-adrenergic receptor agonists, relaxing smooth muscles, including the myometrium. Binding of the receptor activates a cascade of intracellular reactions that affect adenyl cyclase and protein kinase. This cascade decreases the availability of intracellular calcium and the activity of myosin light-chain kinases, thus suppressing myometrial contractility.[30]

The efficacy of beta-mimetics as a tocolytic has predominately involved studies that compared ritodrine with another tocolytic agent or placebo. In a Cochrane meta-analysis of 11 randomized trials of beta-mimetics versus placebo for preterm labor, beta-mimetics decreased the risk of delivery within 48 hours and showed a trend toward reduction in delivery within 7 days, but there was no reduction in preterm birth or neonatal morbidity.[31] Based on the available literature, beta-mimetics do not seem to be a superior tocolytic than other medications. When beta-mimetics were compared with nifedipine in a large meta-analysis of 16 trials, beta-mimetics were not as effective as nifedipine in reducing the risk of delivery within 7 days or before 34 weeks gestation. They were also less effective at reducing the risk for neonatal respiratory distress syndrome.[32] In another review of 5 studies comparing beta-mimetics with magnesium sulfate, beta-mimetics were not associated with reducing delivery at any interval (within 48 hours, 7 days, or before 37 weeks) or in reducing low birth weight infants.[16]

Terbutaline is the most commonly used beta-mimetic for preterm labor in the United States and it is generally administered as a subcutaneous injection. Given its off-label use, the dosing may vary, but, most commonly, 0.25 mg is given subcutaneously and may be repeated in 15 to 30 minutes if there is inadequate response. Total dosing in 4 hours should not exceed 0.5 mg. Common maternal side effects secondary to beta-mimetics include tachycardia, tremor, dyspnea, chest discomfort, palpitations, and hyperglycemia.[8,33] These side effects may be unpleasant to the patient and often result in discontinuation of treatment. More rare side effects include pulmonary edema and myocardial ischemia, but these may be related to other confounding factors, like fluid overload, infection, preeclampsia, or underlying cardiac disease. With prolonged use of beta-mimetics, tachyphylaxis may develop.

Given the known side effects, this class of medication is contraindicated in patients with known cardiac disease or poorly controlled diabetes. It should be withheld if maternal heart rate increases to more than 120 beats/minute or the patient experiences significant symptoms such as dyspnea or chest pain.

Beta-mimetics cross the placental barrier and may lead to fetal effects. Side effects include fetal tachycardia in response to maternal tachycardia and neonatal hypoglycemia linked to maternal hyperglycemia.[34] In addition, question has been raised linking beta-mimetics to an increased risk of neonatal intraventricular hemorrhage,[35,36] although this has been refuted in other studies.[37–39]

CALCIUM CHANNEL BLOCKERS

Calcium channel blockers are typically used in the treatment of hypertension, angina, and coronary artery disease and exert their effect by preventing reuptake of calcium ions via the voltage-dependent calcium channels. The resultant decrease in intracellular calcium leads to inhibition of actin and myosin interaction and, therefore, decreased myometrial contractility.[1,40] Given their ability to relax smooth muscle, calcium channel blockers, in particular nifedipine, are widely used tocolytic agents.

A recent systematic review and meta-analysis of 26 randomized, controlled trials evaluated nifedipine (Procardia) compared with other tocolytics, placebo, or no treatment in the management of preterm labor. To date, no placebo-controlled trials of nifedipine have been published. When compared with beta-mimetics, nifedipine showed a significant reduction in the risk of delivery within 7 days of initiation of treatment (37% vs 45%) as well as a reduction in rate of delivery before 34 weeks

(48% vs 62%). When nifedipine was compared with magnesium sulfate, there was no overall difference in delivery within 48 hours or before 34 or 37 weeks' gestation. This meta-analysis also revealed a significant improvement in neonatal outcomes with nifedipine tocolysis including a reduction in the rate of the common neonatal morbidities of respiratory distress syndrome, necrotizing enterocolitis, and intraventricular hemorrhage. Nifedipine was also associated with fewer NICU admissions and shorter NICU stays.[32]

There are numerous dosing regimens for tocolysis with nifedipine discussed in the literature with most using oral capsules. Initial loading doses range from 10 to 40 mg followed by 10 to 20 mg every 4 to 6 hours, with the dose titrated based on contraction pattern.[32,40] Nifedipine is usually well-tolerated with minimal cardiovascular alterations.[41] In a meta-analysis, nifedipine was less likely to result in maternal side effects when compared with other tocolytics such as beta-mimetics or magnesium sulfate.[32] The majority of maternal side effects with nifedipine are related to relaxation of endothelial smooth muscle, which leads to peripheral vasodilation. Maternal symptoms often include nausea, flushing, headache, dizziness, and palpitations. Peripheral vasodilation leads to a compensatory rise in heart rate and stroke, volume which increases cardiac output, allowing for maintenance of blood pressure in women with no underlying cardiovascular disease. Rare but more serious maternal side effects include pulmonary edema, hypoxia, myocardial infarction, atrial fibrillation, and severe hypotension.[40] Calcium channel blockers should be used with caution in conjunction with magnesium sulfate as cases of cardiovascular collapse have been reported.

The fetal effects of calcium channel blockers are related to its peripheral vasodilative effects and risk of maternal hypotension which can lead to hypoperfusion of the uterus and placenta. Therefore, monitoring of maternal blood pressure and avoidance of calcium channel blockers in women at high risk for hypotension (cardiovascular disease, multiple gestations) are recommended.

PROSTAGLANDIN INHIBITORS

Indomethacin (Indocin), a nonselective COX inhibitor, is the most widely used prostaglandin inhibitor to treat preterm labor. Prostaglandins are known to play a crucial role in the onset of labor through the formation of gap junctions in the myometrium that increase intracellular calcium and facilitate myometrial contractility. Prostaglandin inhibitors function as tocolytics through inhibition of the COX enzyme responsible for converting arachidonic acid to prostaglandins.

Indomethacin has been shown to be an effective tocolytic agent. In addition, it is easy to administer, inexpensive, and has minimal maternal side effects. A 2005 Cochrane review of COX inhibitors for treating preterm labor evaluated 13 trials with a total of 713 women.[42] Indomethacin was shown to be effective when compared with placebo at reducing preterm birth before 37 weeks in 1 trial that included 36 women. In addition, there was a significant increase in gestational age by 3.5 weeks and birth weight of 716 g in 2 trials of 67 women compared with placebo. Despite these findings, there was no difference in perinatal mortality or morbidity, including respiratory distress syndrome or intraventricular hemorrhage. In this same review, 3 trials of 168 women evaluated indomethacin compared with other tocolytic agents, including beta-mimetics and magnesium sulfate. A similar reduction in preterm birth before 37 weeks was seen without any difference in overall perinatal mortality. Selective COX-2 inhibitors such as celecoxib (Celebrex) and rofecoxib (Vioxx) have also been compared with indomethacin with no appreciated difference in maternal or neonatal outcomes.

For tocolytic therapy, indomethacin is generally administered as a loading dose of 50 to 100 mg orally or 50 mg rectally followed by 25 to 50 mg every 6 hours for 48 hours.[43] Maternal side effects are primarily related to the gastrointestinal tract and include nausea, vomiting, gastroesophageal reflux, and gastritis. In addition, platelet dysfunction may occur with use of prostaglandin inhibitors. Selective COX-2 inhibitors have fewer gastrointestinal side effects; however, they are associated with increased cardiovascular risks and, therefore, should be used with caution. Overall, studies have shown that prostaglandin inhibitors are better tolerated and have a lower discontinuation rate owing to side effects than other tocolytics such as beta-mimetics and magnesium sulfate.[42,44]

The usefulness of prostaglandin inhibitors as tocolytics is limited by their effects on the fetus, primarily premature closure of the ductus arteriosus and oligohydramnios. Long-term use of indomethacin is associated with premature closure of the ductus arteriosus in 25% to 50% of pregnancies and results in oligohydramnios in 5% to 70% of pregnancies. A retrospective study of 124 women receiving prolonged indomethacin (≥48 hours) reported the incidence of ductal constriction to be less than previously reported at 6.5% with reversal of constriction 24 to 48 hours after discontinuation of therapy.[45] In addition, the incidence of ductal constriction is reported to be dependent on gestational age at the time of use with increased risk of premature closure at later gestational ages (>31 weeks).[46,47] When used for a short duration (<48 hours), the incidence of oligohydramnios is low. In a study of 61 women before 34 weeks' gestation, the incidence of oligohydramnios was only 3.3% with return to normal amniotic fluid volume within 24 hours of discontinuation.[48] Indomethacin has been linked to other adverse neonatal outcomes, including necrotizing enterocolitis, intraventricular hemorrhage, and cardiac, pulmonary, and renal abnormalities, although these associations were not supported in a more recent meta-analysis of randomized and observational studies.[49] Although concern for fetal side effects of indomethacin may limit prolonged use, it seems to be a safe and effective tocolytic when used for a short period of time.

OXYTOCIN RECEPTOR ANTAGONIST

Given the overall limited efficacy of traditional tocolytic therapy, many European nations have explored the use of an oxytocin receptor antagonist atosiban (Tractocile). Atosiban, in theory, should have limited systemic maternal effects because of its site-specific action on myometrial cells in the uterus and myoepithelial cells in mammary glands, the only known locations of oxytocin receptor expression. Atosiban is a synthetic peptide that functions by blocking oxytocin from binding to its receptor and by downregulating the number of oxytocin receptors, thus decreasing myometrial contractility.[50,51]

Like other tocolytics, there is uncertainty about the efficacy of atosiban as a first-line tocolytic agent. In a meta-analysis that included 2 randomized, controlled trials that compared atosiban with placebo, a small but significant increase in women undelivered at 48 hours was seen in the atosiban group.[52] This result, however, was not seen in a 2005 Cochrane Review of oxytocin receptor antagonists for inhibiting preterm labor.[53] Atosiban was not shown to delay delivery for 48 hours, prevent preterm birth, or improve neonatal outcomes. Atosiban has also not been shown to be superior to other tocolytics. Two small studies have compared atosiban and nifedipine and did not show a difference in efficacy between the 2 medications.[54,55] Given their limited sample sizes, a larger randomized study would be necessary to better compare treatment superiority. Atosiban has been compared with beta-mimetics in large, randomized, controlled trials in Europe, with no difference in tocolytic effectiveness at 48 hours or 7 days or in neonatal outcomes.[56,57]

Atosiban is administered as a continuous intravenous infusion with a loading dose of 6.75 mg followed by a maintenance dose of 300 μg/min for 3 hours, and then 100 μg/min for up to 48 hours.[57]

Studies of atosiban show limited side effects on both mother and fetus. When administered intravenously, it achieves a rapid maternal plasma steady state followed by a high clearance rate, with an estimated half-life of 18 minutes.[58] In addition, studies suggest that atosiban crosses the placenta in a limited fashion and does not seem to accumulate in the fetal circulation.[59] Unlike some tocolytics, atosiban does not alter maternal or fetal cardiovascular parameters in animal models, making it a very tolerable drug.[60] The most commonly cited maternal adverse reactions to atosiban include headache, nausea, and vomiting (8%–12%).[61] These adverse effects are more common during the loading period of the drug and decrease significantly during the maintenance period of the infusion.[62] In terms of overall maternal side effects, studies comparing atosiban with nifedipine and beta-mimetics favor atosiban.[54–56,61]

Questions have been raised about higher rates of death among infants exposed to atosiban. In a study by Romero and colleageus[63] that included 583 infants, more women were unexpectedly randomly allocated to receive atosiban as opposed to placebo before 26 weeks' gestation (10% vs 5%). There were more fetal–infant deaths in the group receiving atosiban (4.5% vs 1.7%). Seven of the 10 infant deaths in the atosiban group were among babies weighing less than 650 g; therefore, extreme prematurity may have played a significant role in the adverse neonatal outcomes in this group.[63,64] Given the increased infant deaths in the atosiban group, the US Food and Drug Administration has not approved the use of this drug for tocolysis in the United States.[30]

SUMMARY

The pathophysiology leading to preterm labor is not well understood and often multifactorial; initiating factors include intrauterine infection, inflammation, ischemia, overdistension, and hemorrhage.[3] Given these different potential causes, directing therapy for preterm labor has been difficult and suboptimal. To date, no single drug has been identified as successful in treating all of the underlying mechanisms leading to preterm labor. In addition, the methodology of many of the tocolytic studies is limited by lack of sufficient patient numbers, lack of comparison with a placebo, and inconsistent use of glucocorticoids. The limitations in these individual studies make it difficult to evaluate the efficacy of a single tocolytic by meta-analysis. Despite these limitations, the goals for tocolysis for preterm labor are clear: To complete a course of glucocorticoids and secure the appropriate level of neonatal care for the fetus in the event of preterm delivery.

The literature demonstrates that many tocolytic agents inhibit uterine contractility. The decision as to which tocolytic agent should be used as first-line therapy for a patient is based on multiple factors, including gestational age, the patient's medical history, common and severe side effects, and a patient's response to therapy. In a patient at less than 32 weeks gestation, indomethacin may be a reasonable first choice based on its efficacy, ease of administration, and minimal side effects. Concurrent administration of magnesium for neuroprotection may be given. At 32 to 34 weeks, nifedipine may be a reasonable first choice because it does not carry the fetal risks of indomethacin at these later gestational ages, is easy to administer, and has limited side effects relative to beta-mimetics.

In an effort to review a commonly faced obstetrical complication, this article has provided a summary of the most commonly used tocolytics, their mechanisms of action, side effects, and clinical data regarding their efficacy.

REFERENCES

1. Blumenfeld Y, Lyell D. Prematurity prevention: the role of acute tocolysis. Curr Opin Obstet Gynecol 2009;21:136–41.
2. Roos C, Scheepers LH, Bloemenkamp KW, et al. Assessment of perinatal outcome after sustained tocolysis in early labour (APOSTEL-II trial). BMC Pregnancy Childbirth 2009;9:42.
3. Goldenberg RL, Culhane JF, Iams JD, et al. Epidemiology and causes of preterm birth. Lancet 2008;371:75–84.
4. Mercer BM, Goldenberg RL, Moawad AH, et al. The preterm prediction study: effect of gestational age and cause of preterm birth on subsequent obstetric outcome. National Institute of Child Health and Human Development Maternal-Fetal Medicine Units Network. Am J Obstet Gynecol 1999;181:1216–21.
5. da Fonseca EB, Bittar RE, Carvalho MH, et al. Prophylactic administration of progesterone by vaginal suppository to reduce the incidence of spontaneous preterm birth in women at increased risk: a randomized placebo-controlled double-blind study. Am J Obstet Gynecol 2003;188:419.
6. Meis PJ, Klebanoff M, Thom E, et al. Prevention of recurrent preterm delivery by 17 alpha-hydroxyprogesterone caproate. N Engl J Med 2003;348:2379–85.
7. Goldenberg RL, Hauth JC, Andrews WW. Intrauterine infection and preterm delivery. N Engl J Med 2000;342:1500–7.
8. Gyetvai K, Hannah ME, Hodnett ED, et al. Tocolytics for preterm labor: a systematic review. Obstet Gynecol 1999;94:869–77.
9. Macones GA, Bader TJ, Asch DA. Optimising maternal-fetal outcomes in preterm labour: a decision analysis. Br J Obstet Gynaecol 1998;105:541–50.
10. Morgan MA, Goldenberg RL, Schulkin J. Obstetrician-gynecologists' screening and management of preterm birth. Obstet Gynecol 2008;112:35–41.
11. Steer CM, Petrie RH. A comparison of magnesium sulfate and alcohol for the prevention of premature labor. Am J Obstet Gynecol 1977;129:1–4.
12. Elin RJ. Magnesium: the fifth but forgotten electrolyte. Am J Clin Pathol 1994;102:616–22.
13. Wolf FI, Torsello A, Fasanella S, et al. Cell physiology of magnesium. Mol Aspects Med 2003;24:11–26.
14. Fomin VP, Gibbs SG, Vanam R, et al. Effect of magnesium sulfate on contractile force and intracellular calcium concentration in pregnant human myometrium. Am J Obstet Gynecol 2006;194:1384–90.
15. Phillippe M. Cellular mechanisms underlying magnesium sulfate inhibition of phasic myometrial contractions. Biochem Biophys Res Commun 1998;252:502–7.
16. Mercer BM, Merlino AA, Society for Maternal-Fetal Medicine. Magnesium sulfate for preterm labor and preterm birth. Obstet Gynecol 2009;114:650–68.
17. Simhan HN, Caritis S. Inhibition of acute preterm labor. Available at: http://www.uptodate.com/contents/inhibition-of-acute-preterm-labor. Accessed December 8, 2011.
18. Terrone DA, Rinehart BK, Kimmel ES, et al. A prospective, randomized, controlled trial of high and low maintenance doses of magnesium sulfate for acute tocolysis. Am J Obstet Gynecol 2000;182:1477–82.

19. Lyell DJ, Pullen K, Campbell L, et al. Magnesium sulfate compared with nifedipine for acute tocolysis of preterm labor: a randomized controlled trial. Obstet Gynecol 2007;110:61–7.
20. Twickler DM, McIntire DD, Alexander JM, et al. Effects of magnesium sulfate on preterm fetal cerebral blood flow using Doppler analysis: a randomized controlled trial. Obstet Gynecol 2010;115:21–5.
21. Lipsitz PJ. The clinical and biochemical effects of excess magnesium in the newborn. Pediatrics 1971;47:501–9.
22. Crowther CA, Hiller JE, Doyle LW. Magnesium sulphate for preventing preterm birth in threatened preterm labour. Cochrane Database Syst Rev 2002;4:CD001060.
23. Crowther CA, Hiller JE, Doyle LW, et al. Effect of magnesium sulfate given for neuroprotection before preterm birth: a randomized controlled trial. JAMA 2003;290:2669–76.
24. Marret S, Marpeau L, Bénichou J. Benefit of magnesium sulfate given before very preterm birth to protect infant brain. Pediatrics 2008;121:225–6.
25. Rouse DJ, Hirtz DG, Thom E, et al. A randomized, controlled trial of magnesium sulfate for the prevention of cerebral palsy. N Engl J Med 2008;359:895–905.
26. Wesselius-de Casparis A, Thiery M, Yo le Sian A, et al. Results of double-blind, multicentre study with ritodrine in premature labour. Br Med J 1971;3:144–7.
27. Walters WA, Wood C. A trial of oral ritodrine for the prevention of premature labour. Br J Obstet Gynaecol 1977;84:26–30.
28. Lauersen NH, Merkatz IR, Tejani N, et al. Inhibition of premature labor: a multicenter comparison of ritodrine and ethanol. Am J Obstet Gynecol 1977;127:837–45.
29. Terbutaline: label change: warning against use for treatment of preterm labor. Available at: http://www.fda.gov/Safety/MedWatch/SafetyInformation/SafetyAlertsfor HumanMedicalProducts/ucm243843.htm.
30. Simhan HN, Caritis SN. Prevention of preterm delivery. N Engl J Med 2007;357:477–87.
31. Anotayanonth S, Subhedar NV, Garner P, et al. Betamimetics for inhibiting preterm labour. Cochrane Database Syst Rev 2004;4:CD004352.
32. Conde-Agudelo A, Romero R, Kusanovic JP. Nifedipine in the management of preterm labor: a systematic review and metaanalysis. Am J Obstet Gynecol 2011;204:134.e1–20.
33. Caritis SN, Toig G, Heddinger LA, et al. A double-blind study comparing ritodrine and terbutaline in the treatment of preterm labor. Am J Obstet Gynecol 1984;150:7–14.
34. Golichowski AM, Hathaway DR, Fineberg N, et al. Tocolytic and hemodynamic effects of nifedipine in the ewe. Am J Obstet Gynecol 1985;151:1134–40.
35. Groome LJ, Goldenberg RL, Cliver SP, et al. Neonatal periventricular-intraventricular hemorrhage after maternal beta-sympathomimetic tocolysis. The March of Dimes Multicenter Study Group. Am J Obstet Gynecol 1992;167:873–9.
36. Papatsonis DN, Kok JH, van Geijn HP, et al. Neonatal effects of nifedipine and ritodrine for preterm labor. Obstet Gynecol 2000;95:477–81.
37. Weintraub Z, Solovechick M, Reichman B, et al. Effect of maternal tocolysis on the incidence of severe periventricular/intraventricular haemorrhage in very low birth-weight infants. Arch Dis Child Fetal Neonatal Ed 2001;85:F13–7.
38. Ozcan T, Turan C, Ekici E, et al. Ritodrine tocolysis and neonatal intraventricular-periventricular hemorrhage. Gynecol Obstet Invest 1995;39:60–2.
39. Palta M, Sadek M, Lim TS, et al. Association of tocolytic therapy with antenatal steroid administration and infant outcomes. Newborn Lung Project. Am J Perinatol 1998;15:87–92.

40. Nassar AH, Aoun J, Usta IM. Calcium channel blockers for the management of preterm birth: a review. Am J Perinatol 2011;28:57–66.

41. Ferguson JE 2nd, Dyson DC, Holbrook RH Jr, et al. Cardiovascular and metabolic effects associated with nifedipine and ritodrine tocolysis. Am J Obstet Gynecol 1989;161:788–95.

42. King J, Flenady V, Cole S, et al. Cyclo-oxygenase (COX) inhibitors for treating preterm labour. Cochrane Database Syst Rev 2005:CD001992.

43. ACOG Practice Bulletin No. 43: Management of preterm labor. Obstet Gynecol 2003;101:1039–47.

44. Haas DM, Imperiale TF, Kirkpatrick PR, et al. Tocolytic therapy: a meta-analysis and decision analysis. Am J Obstet Gynecol 2009;113:585–94.

45. Savage AH, Anderson BL, Simhan HN. The safety of prolonged indomethacin therapy. Am J Perinatol 2007;24:207–13.

46. Moise KJ Jr, Huhta JC, Sharif DS, et al. Indomethacin in the treatment of premature labor. Effects on the fetal ductus arteriosus. N Engl J Med 1988;319:327–31.

47. Vermillion ST, Scardo JA, Lashus AG, et al. The effect of indomethacin tocolysis on fetal ductus arteriosus constriction with advancing gestational age. Am J Obstet Gynecol 1997;177:256–61.

48. Sandruck JC, Grobman WA, Gerber SE. The effect of short-term indomethacin therapy on amniotic fluid volume. Am J Obstet Gynecol 2005;192:1443–5.

49. Loe SM, Sanchez-Ramos L, Kaunitz AM. Assessing the neonatal safety of indomethacin tocolysis: a systematic review with meta-analysis. Obstet Gynecol 2005;106:173–9.

50. Akerlund M, Carlsson AM, Melin P, et al. The effect on the human uterus of two newly developed competitive inhibitors of oxytocin and vasopressin. Acta Obstet Gynecol Scand 1985;64:499–504.

51. Engstrøm T, Bratholm P, Vilhardt H, et al. Effect of oxytocin receptor and beta2-adrenoceptor blockade on myometrial oxytocin receptors in parturient rats. Biol Reprod 1999;60:322–9.

52. Coomarasamy A, Knox EM, Gee H, et al. Oxytocin antagonists for tocolysis in preterm labour: a systematic review. Med Sci Monit 2002;8:RA268–73.

53. Papatsonis D, Flenady V, Cole S, et al. Oxytocin receptor antagonists for inhibiting preterm labour. Cochrane Database Syst Rev 2005;3:CD004452.

54. Al-Omari WR, Al-Shammaa HB, Al-Tikriti EM, et al. Atosiban and nifedipine in acute tocolysis: a comparative study. Eur J Obstet Gynecol Reprod Biol 2006;128:129–34.

55. Kashanian M, Akbarian AR, Soltanzadeh M. Atosiban and nifedipine for the treatment of preterm labor. Int J Gynaecol Obstet 2005;91:10–4.

56. European atosiban Study Group. The oxytocin antagonist atosiban versus the beta-agonist terbutaline in the treatment of preterm labor. A randomized, double-blind, controlled study. Acta Obstet Gynecol Scand 2001;80:413–22.

57. Worldwide Atosiban versus Beta-agonists Study Group. Effectiveness and safety of the oxytocin antagonist atosiban versus beta-adrenergic agonists in the treatment of preterm labour. BJOG 2001;108:133.

58. Goodwin TM, Millar L, North L, et al. The pharmacokinetics of the oxytocin antagonist atosiban in pregnant women with preterm uterine contractions. Am J Obstet Gynecol 1995;173:913–7.

59. Valenzuela GJ, Craig J, Bernhardt MD, et al. Placental passage of the oxytocin antagonist atosiban. Am J Obstet Gynecol 1995;172:1304–6.

60. Greig PC, Massmann GA, Demarest KT, et al. Maternal and fetal cardiovascular effects and placental transfer of the oxytocin antagonist atosiban in late-gestation pregnant sheep. Am J Obstet Gynecol 1993;169:897–902.

61. Moutquin JM, Sherman D, Cohen H, et al. Double-blind, randomized, controlled trial of atosiban and ritodrine in the treatment of preterm labor: a multicenter effectiveness and safety study. Am J Obstet Gynecol 2000;182:1191–9.
62. Goodwin TM, Valenzuela G, Silver H, et al. Treatment of preterm labor with the oxytocin antagonist atosiban. Am J Perinatol 1996;13:143–6.
63. Romero R, Sibai BM, Sanchez-Ramos L, et al. An oxytocin receptor antagonist (atosiban) in the treatment of preterm labor: a randomized, double-blind, placebo-controlled trial with tocolytic rescue. Am J Obstet Gynecol 2000;182:1173–83.
64. de Heus R, Mulder EJ, Visser GH. Management of preterm labor: atosiban or nifedipine? Int J Womens Health 2010;2:137–42.

Early Term Births: Considerations in Management

Luisa Wetta, MD*, Alan T.N. Tita, MD, PhD

KEYWORDS

- Early term birth • Fetal lung maturity • Maternal outcomes
- Neonatal outcomes

It is often said that the 2 key decisions that obstetricians routinely make address the questions: When is the best time to deliver? and Through what mode should the delivery be undertaken? Ideally, delivery should occur at term. Traditionally, "term birth" refers to any birth between 37 weeks and 0 days of gestation and 41 weeks and 6 days. However, data suggesting heterogeneity in outcomes within this group has led many to reconsider the definition of a "term birth."[1] As a result, term births may be subgrouped into 2 categories, "early" term births and "full" term births. Early term births encompass neonates born between 37 and 0/7 weeks gestation and 38 6/7 weeks gestation; full-term deliveries are those that occur between 39 and 0/7 weeks gestation and 41 6/7 weeks gestation (births occurring beyond this period are postdate or postterm).[1,2] Some providers and patients may assume that optimal outcomes occur uniformly "at term," whereas births at 37 or 38 weeks are associated with worse outcomes compared with those at 39 to 40 weeks. Therefore, the "early term" designation draws appropriate attention to the potential for adverse outcomes and the need to carefully consider the indication for delivery at term but before 39 weeks. Although early term deliveries occurring spontaneously or that are necessary to avoid maternal or fetal complications are unavoidable, it is important to limit the frequency of early births by induction or scheduled cesarean without medical or obstetric reasons. These births contribute to the rising rate of induction and cesarean delivery in the United States and to the ongoing reduction in mean gestational age at delivery. For example, the rates of cesarean delivery in the United States rose from 20.7% in 1996 to 31.8% in 2007,[3] and this number is expected to continue to increase. A main reason for this increase is an increase in the number of primary cesareans and the decline in a trial of labor after cesarean.[4–6] Inductions of labor have

The authors have nothing to disclose.

Maternal and Fetal Medicine Division, UAB Department of Obstetrics & Gynecology, 1700 6th Avenue South, Women & Infants Center, Room 10270, Birmingham, AL 35233, USA

* Corresponding author.

E-mail address: luisa.wetta@obgyn.uab.edu

Obstet Gynecol Clin N Am 39 (2012) 89–97

doi:10.1016/j.ogc.2011.12.002

0889-8545/12/$ – see front matter © 2012 Elsevier Inc. All rights reserved.

obgyn.theclinics.com

Table 1
Incidence of early terms births

Study	Population	% Early Term	% Early Term Among Term Births
Tita et al, 2009[8]	Elective repeat cesarean delivery enrolled at 19 US centers	35.8	35.8
Bailit et al, 2010[10]	Singleton pregnancies, 10 US centers, 34–42 weeks	—	31.5[a]
Clark et al, 2010[10]	27 US hospitals, deliveries	36.8	43.8 (2007)–29.3 (2009)
Reddy et a, 2011[2]	US Singleton live births from 1995 to 2006	25.3	30.7
Wilmink et al, 2010[11]	Elective cesarean delivery in The Netherlands perinatal registry	56.6	56.6

[a] Calculated from data presented in Bailit et al,[10] **Table 2.**

also increased in the United States, from 9.5% in 1990 to 22.5% in 2006.[3] A significant proportion of these inductions and cesareans are elective,[7] and may even be scheduled solely for patient or provider convenience.

PREVALENCE AND SUBTYPES

The frequency of early term births naturally varies widely by patient characteristics, provider practice patterns, and health system factors.[2,8–11] These births fall into 3 main categories: Those that are spontaneous (and therefore inevitable), those that are medically or obstetrically indicated to improve maternal or fetal outcomes, and those that are performed without obvious medical or obstetric justification (so-called elective deliveries). Obstetric indications are numerous and include preeclampsia or gestational hypertension, nonreassuring fetal heart tones, premature rupture of membranes, placenta previa, abruption, and prior classical cesarean with attendant risk of rupture with labor.

Table 1 presents the prevalence of early term births for various study populations. In 1 large, US study of presumed elective cesarean deliveries, more than one third were performed before 39 weeks.[8] An even higher number of elective cesareans (>50%), were performed before 39 weeks in a Dutch cohort.[11]

NEONATAL OUTCOMES

The available data reveal increased respiratory morbidities in neonates born at 37 or 38 completed weeks of gestation compared with those born after 39 weeks (**Table 2**), suggesting a continuum with late preterm births. Overall, the risks increase progressively as gestational age at birth declines.[2,8,9,11–14] Recent studies suggest that increased morbidity with earlier delivery at term is not limited to the respiratory system.

A large study by the Maternal-Fetal Medicine Units Network network[8] examined the association between delivery before 39 weeks and the risk of adverse neonatal outcomes among women who underwent a repeat cesarean without labor or obvious maternal or fetal indications for delivery (elective delivery). Neonatal outcomes that were studied included death, adverse respiratory outcomes including respiratory

Table 2
Odds ratios of respiratory morbidities and neonatal intensive care unit in early term versus full-term neonates delivered by elective repeat cesarean

	37 Weeks	38 Weeks	39 Weeks	40 Weeks
Respiratory distress syndrome				
Tita et al, 2009[8]	4.2 (2.7–6.6)	2.1 (1.5–2.9)	Reference	1.1 (0.6–2.0)
Wilmink et al, 2010[11]	3.8 (1.4–10.5)	1.9 (0.8–4.5)	—	—
Transient tachypnea of the newborn				
Tita et al, 2009[8]	1.8 (1.2–2.5)	1.5 (1.2–1.9)	Reference	0.9 (0.6–1.3)
Wilmink et al, 2010[11]	2.9 (2.1–3.9)	1.8 (1.4–2.3)	Reference	1.0 (0.6–1.6)
Neonatal intensive care admission				
Tita et al, 2009[8]	2.3 (1.9–3.0)	1.5 (1.3–1.7)	Reference	0.8 (0.6–1.0)
Wilmink et al, 2010[11]	2.8 (1.3–5.8)	1.3 (0.7–2.3)		0.5 (0.1–2.4)

Data are presented as odds ratios with 95% confidence intervals relative to 39 weeks.

distress syndrome or transient tachypnea of the newborn, hypoglycemia, newborn sepsis, confirmed seizures, necrotizing enterocolitis, hypoxic–ischemic encephalopathy, cardiopulmonary resuscitation or ventilator support within 24 hours after birth, umbilical cord pH below 7.0, a 5-minute Apgar score of 3 or below, admission to the neonatal intensive care unit, or prolonged hospitalization (≥5 days). The primary outcome was a composite of neonatal death and any of the adverse outcomes described above. Of the 24,077 repeat cesarean deliveries at term, 13,258 (52%) were performed electively. Compared with births at 39 weeks, births at 37 and 38 weeks were associated with an increased risk of the primary outcome. The risk of adverse respiratory outcomes, mechanical ventilations, newborn sepsis, hypoglycemia, admission to the neonatal intensive care unit, and hospitalization for 5 days or more was also increased (2- to 4-fold at 37 weeks and 1.5- to 2-fold at 38 weeks).[8] Importantly, about 52% of all early term births occurred within the 3 days before 39 0/7 weeks, and these births were also associated with increased neonatal morbidity compared with births at 39 completed weeks.[8]

A study by Wilmink and co-workers[11] in 2010 examined The Netherlands birth registry to study similar outcomes to the ones described by Tita and colleagues (MFMU).[8] They examined 20,973 elective cesarean deliveries; the primary outcome was a composite of neonatal morbidity and mortality, including respiratory morbidities, sepsis, metabolic complications, neurologic dysfunction, and neonatal intensive care admissions. Results also showed that infants born before 39 weeks were at a higher risk of morbidity and mortality. The absolute risks in this study were 20.6% at 37 weeks, 12.5% before 38 weeks, 9.5% at 39 weeks, and 9.4% at 40 weeks.[11]

Clark and colleagues[10] examined the impact of deliveries at less than 39 weeks gestation on the rates of stillbirth and neonatal intensive care admissions. In this review of 27 US hospitals, 36.8% of all births (vaginal and cesarean) occurred at greater than or equal to 37 weeks gestation. Of all births at greater than 37 weeks, 43.8% occurred between 37 0/7 and 38 6/7 completed weeks. Overall, 9.6% of all deliveries between 37 0/7 and 38 6/7 weeks were elective and 8.9% of neonatal intensive care admissions were to births occurring at or greater than 37 0/7 weeks of gestation. After implantation of strategies to prevent elective term deliveries, the elective term delivery rate declined from 9.6% to 4.3% and the rate of neonatal intensive care admissions beyond 37 weeks fell by 16%.[10]

Reddy and co-workers[2] examined racial and ethnic differences between early term and full-term infants. This study also supported findings from previous studies that early term infants have higher neonatal mortality rates that extend into the postneonatal and infant periods. At 37 and 38 weeks compared with 40 weeks of gestation, mortality rates were increased. There was also a racial disparity in these mortality rates, with Blacks having the highest rates, and Hispanics have the lowest rates, compared with Caucasians.[2]

It is well-established that preterm birth is among the strongest predictors of cerebral palsy, with the risk increasing as gestational age at delivery decreases. However, studies have shown that a majority of infants born with cerebral palsy are delivered after 36 weeks' gestation.[15] Moster and associates[16] conducted a population-based study of the birth registry of Norway and found that, compared with delivery at 40 weeks' gestation, delivery at 37 or 38 weeks gestation was associated with an increased risk of cerebral palsy.[16]

An increase in the cumulative risk of fetal demise with advancing gestational age may be preventable by early delivery. This is a major reason early delivery is indicated for high-risk conditions. However, for otherwise healthy pregnancies the increase in risk with each additional week is so small that it does not seem to outweigh the risks of early delivery. In fact, stillbirth rates did not increase significantly after interventions to reduce the rates of early delivery.[10]

Lung Maturity Testing and Outcomes

Current American College of Obstetricians and Gynecologists' guidelines allow delivery before 39 weeks if fetal lung maturity demonstrated.[17] Documentation of fetal lung maturity in theory should reduce the neonatal risk of respiratory morbidity. Fetal lung maturity testing may be accomplished by both invasive and noninvasive methods. Noninvasive methods to determine a term pregnancy are based on ultrasound dating, the duration of a positive pregnancy test, and the duration of time since the first fetal heart tones were first recorded by Doppler or by a fetoscope. If ultrasound dating performed before 12 weeks of gestation supports a gestational age of at least 39 weeks or ultrasound dating performed between 12 and 20 weeks supports a clinically determined gestational age (based on last menstrual period) of greater than or equal to 39 weeks, lung maturity is inferred. Alternatively, a positive pregnancy test must have been obtained for at least 36 weeks and fetal heart tones must have been recorded for at least 30 weeks by Doppler ultrasonography or 24 weeks by a fetoscope. The use of noninvasive methods generally prevents early term or preterm birth.[17,18]

An amniocentesis is the basis for most invasive tests to determine fetal lung maturity. Several tests are widely utilized for determination of lung maturation, depending on physician preference, availability, and presence or absence of contaminants.[17] Examples of these tests include surfactant/albumin ratio (TDx-FLM II, Abbott, Abbott Park, IL), the lecithin/sphingomyelin ratio, phosphatidylglycerol, lamellar body count, optical density at 650 nm, and the foam stability index. Interpretation of these tests, however, may be influenced by several different factors, including gestational age, the presence of blood or meconium, oligohydramnios or polyhydramnios, or the presence of maternal diabetes.[17]

Although FLM before delivery reduces respiratory morbidity compared with gestational age–matched cohorts, morbidity is not reduced to the levels obtained at 39 to 40 weeks. Furthermore, other neonatal morbidities are also increased. A large study examined neonatal outcomes after fetal lung maturity had been demonstrated.[19] This retrospective cohort study examined women delivered between 36 and 38 and 6/7 weeks' gestation after positive fetal lung maturity testing. The primary outcome was a composite of death, adverse respiratory outcomes, hypoglycemia, treated hyperbilirubinemia, generalized seizures, necrotizing enterocolitis, hypoxic ischemic encephalopathy, periventricular leukomalacia, and suspected or proven sepsis. Despite confirmation of fetal lung maturity, infants delivered at 36 to 38 weeks had significantly higher risks of adverse outcomes compared with those delivered at 39 to 40 weeks gestation.[19]

A larger study of more than 10,000 deliveries showed similar results regarding confirmation of fetal lung maturity. Neonates delivered between 36 and 38 weeks gestation after confirmation of fetal lung maturity had a respiratory morbidity rate of 7.3% compared with 1.6% among those delivered after 39 weeks. Admission to neonatal intensive care unit was also more common in those delivered early term after demonstrated lung maturity (9.6% vs 3.2%).[20]

MATERNAL OUTCOMES

As shown, early term births are associated with increased respiratory and other neonatal morbidities and the increased risks persist despite positive fetal lung maturity testing before delivery. Concerning the impact of early delivery on maternal morbidity and mortality, is there a maternal benefit to delivery before 39 weeks' gestation that may outweigh neonatal risks?

Limited data exist on maternal morbidity and mortality related to early term deliveries. Information on elective repeat cesarean deliveries before 39 weeks does not support a maternal benefit to early delivery and suggests an increase in health care costs related to an increased duration of maternal hospitalization. Among elective repeat cesarean deliveries, there were no differences in maternal morbidities between delivery at 39 weeks and delivery in the early term period (37 to 38 weeks).[21] Maternal outcomes examined included death, uterine rupture, need for hysterectomy, transfusion, infections, and anesthetic and surgical complications. However, women delivered in the early term period were more likely to have prolonged hospitalization (>4 days), most likely owing to prolonged hospitalization of their newborns. A report on examining selected maternal outcomes (endometritis, hysterectomy, intensive care admission, and length of hospital stay) by mode of labor onset and gestational age did not associate early term delivery with improved maternal outcomes.[9]

Overall, existing studies do not suggest a maternal benefit to elective early term delivery. However, few studies exist that have examined maternal outcomes in relation to gestational age. Therefore, additional studies are warranted to further elucidate the relationship between maternal mortality/morbidity and early term deliveries.

MANAGEMENT

Because early term pregnancies represent a continuum with late preterm births, similar principles of management apply. An outline of the key considerations include the following. The primary objective remains to attain optimal outcomes for both the fetus and the mother, ideally through delivery at 39 0/7 weeks or later in the absence of high-risk complications. The risks of delivery at less than 39 weeks must be weighed against the risks of continuing pregnancy (eg, fetal demise, adverse maternal or perinatal outcomes related to pregnancy complications such as abruption, bleeding previa, preeclampsia, or membrane rupture). Acceptably, there may circumstances where the absence or the presence of indications for delivery may not be clear cut.

Box 1
Selected indications for delivery at <39 weeks

Absolutely contraindicated

  Patient desire or convenience

  Provider desire or convenience

Absolutely indicated

  Gestational hypertension

  Preeclampsia

  Nonreassuring fetal testing

  Abruption

  History of prior classical cesarean section

  History of a prior myomectomy

  Oligohydramnios

  Fetal growth restriction with oligohydramnios

  Preterm premature rupture of membranes

  Chorioamnionitis

  Monochorionic monoamniotic twins

Controversial

  Chronic hypertension (controlled)

  Diabetes mellitus (controlled)

  Multiple gestations

  Intrauterine growth retardation without oligohydramnios

  Fetal congenital malformations

For some conditions, where there is not an acute need to deliver, the optimal timing of delivery remains controversial (uncomplicated twins, well-controlled chronic hypertension, well-controlled diabetes, isolated suspected intrauterine growth retardation). Some have argued that chronic hypertension should be delivered at 38 weeks.[22,23] The default is to attain 39 weeks; still, the careful consideration of other circumstances by the provider could justify earlier delivery. Some situations for which timing of delivery may be controversial are listed **(Box 1)**. A recent expert commentary has provided consensus recommendations concerning the optimal gestational age to deliver women with various conditions.[24] Some examples are:

- Multiple gestations
  - Dichorionic–diamniotic: 38 weeks
  - Monochorionic–diamniotic: 34–37 weeks
  - Monochorionic–monoamniotic: 32–34 weeks
- Chronic hypertension
  - No medications: 38–39 weeks
  - Controlled on medication: 37–39 weeks
  - Difficult to control on medications: 36–37 weeks
  - Gestational hypertension: 38 weeks.

Induction of labor or cesarean delivery performed with or without confirmation of fetal lung maturity, either out of patient or provider convenience, may pose the most threat to public health if allowed unabated. Therefore, it is important to educate both patients and providers on these implications of early term births, especially those that are elective. The American College of Obstetricians and Gynecologists recommends that no elective induction or cesarean delivery be performed before 39 weeks unless there is a clinical indication or documentation of fetal lung maturity.[6,17] Also, the National Quality Forum and the Joint Commission has requested reporting of all deliveries that are electively performed before 39 weeks' gestation.[25]

PREVENTION

Traditionally, patients and providers may perceive "term" births beyond 37 weeks' gestation to be associated with similar and minimal risks to the neonate. A recent survey showed that many women believed that it is safe to deliver before 39 weeks' gestation.[26] Therefore, increased awareness of both providers and patients of the morbidity associated with early term births may enhance prevention.

Some groups have taken action to increase awareness of the situation with the goal of preventing perinatal and infant morbidity and mortality. One such group is the Ohio Perinatal Quality Collorative.[27] This collaborative is composed of 20 Ohio maternity hospitals that account for greater than 47% of the total births in the state of Ohio. The goal of this group was to monitor the indications for delivery among women delivered between 36 0/7 weeks' gestation and 38 6/7 weeks' gestation through program self-reporting. Education and feedback was provided to the participating centers. As a result of this initiative, the rate of scheduled births between 36 0/7 weeks and 38 6/7 weeks without a documented medical indication declined from 25% to less than 5% over a 14-month period.[27]

Similar programs have been established in other centers across the United States.[28] For example, a health care system in Utah initiated a set of guidelines and a system of tracking to discourage early term deliveries. As a result, the prevalence of early term elective deliveries declined from 28% to less than 3% after 6 years.[28] Similar guidelines for elective inductions were implemented at another institution, resulting in an overall decrease in the induction rate, specifically inappropriate elective inductions.[29] Although these efforts should be lauded, it is important to emphasize that they should not prevent providers from proceeding with early delivery when absolutely indicated for maternal or fetal reasons.

SUMMARY

The frequency of early term birth varies depending on patient, provider, and system characteristics. Early term deliveries are associated with suboptimal neonatal outcomes without evidence of maternal benefit. Some early term births are either unavoidable or absolutely indicated for maternal and/or fetal benefit in the setting of medical or obstetric risks. Demonstrated fetal lung maturity before early term birth reduces the risk of respiratory and other morbidities relative to gestational age–matched counterparts but may not reduce the risks to the low levels at 39 to 40 weeks. For some risk situations, it remains controversial whether earlier delivery is beneficial. The assessment of the provider and patient's desires should direct care. In the absence of any obstetric or medical risks, early term delivery should be avoided. A simple intervention that includes administrative support, review of indications, and feedback to providers can dramatically reduce the frequency of early term births over time.

REFERENCES

1. Fleischman AR, Oinuma M, Clark SL. Rethinking the definition of "term pregnancy." Obstet Gynecol 2010;116:136–9.
2. Reddy UM, Bettegowda VR, Dias T, et al. Term pregnancy: a period of heterogeneous risk for infant mortality. Obstet Gynecol 2011;117:1279–87.
3. Martin JA, Hamilton BE, Sutton PD, et al. Births: final data for 2007. Natl Vital Stat Rep 2010;58:1–85.
4. MacDorman M, Declercq E, Menacker F. Recent trends and patterns in cesarean and vaginal birth after cesarean (VBAC) deliveries in the United States. Clin Perinatol 2011;38:179–92.
5. Menacker F, Declercq E, Macdorman MF. Cesarean delivery: background, trends, and epidemiology. Semin Perinatol 2006;30:235–41.
6. American College of Obstetricians and Gynecologists. ACOG Committee Opinion No. 394, December 2007. Cesarean delivery on maternal request. Obstet Gynecol 2007;110:1501.
7. Rayburn WF, Zhang J. Rising rates of labor induction: present concerns and future strategies. Obstet Gynecol 2002;100:164–7.
8. Tita AT, Landon MB, Spong CY, et al; Eunice Kennedy Shriver NICHD Maternal-Fetal Medicine Units Network. Timing of elective repeat cesarean delivery at term and neonatal outcomes. N Engl J Med 2009;360:111–20.
9. Bailit JL, Gregory KD, Reddy UM, et al. Maternal and neonatal outcomes by labor onset type and gestational age. Am J Obstet Gynecol 2010;202:245,e1–245.
10. Clark SL, Frye DR, Meyers JA, et al. Reduction in elective delivery at <39 weeks of gestation: comparative effectiveness of 3 approaches to change and the impact on neonatal intensive care admission and stillbirth. Am J Obstet Gynecol 2010;203:449,e1–6.
11. Wilmink FA, Hukkelhoven CW, Lunshof S, et al. Neonatal outcome following elective cesarean section beyond 37 weeks of gestation: a 7-year retrospective analysis of a national registry. Am J Obstet Gynecol 2010;202:250,e1–8.
12. Morrison JJ, Rennie JM, Milton PJ. Neonatal respiratory morbidity and mode of delivery at term: influence of timing of elective caesarean section. Br J Obstet Gynaecol 1995;102:101–6.
13. Zanardo V, Simbi AK, Franzoi M, et al. Neonatal respiratory morbidity risk and mode of delivery at term: influence of timing of elective caesarean delivery. Acta Paediatr 2004;93:643–7.
14. Engle WA, Kominiarek MA. Late preterm infants, early term infants, and timing of elective deliveries. Clin Perinatol 2008;35:325–41.
15. Moster D, Lie RT, Markestad T. Long-term medical and social consequences of preterm birth. N Engl J Med 2008;359:262–73.
16. Moster D, Wilcox AJ, Vollset SE, et al. Cerebral palsy among term and postterm births. Jama 2010;304:976–82.
17. American College of Obstetricians and Gynecologists. ACOG Committee Opinion: Committee on Obstetrics: Maternal and Fetal Medicine. Number 98: Fetal maturity assessment prior to elective repeat cesarean delivery. September 1991 (replaces No. 77, January 1990). Int J Gynaecol Obstet 1992;38:327.
18. American College of Obstetricians and Gynecologists. ACOG Practice Bulletin No. 107: Induction of labor. ACOG Committee on Practice Bulletins: Obstetrics. Obstet Gynecol 2009;114:386–97.
19. Bates E, Rouse DJ, Mann ML, et al. Neonatal outcomes after demonstrated fetal lung maturity before 39 weeks of gestation. Obstet Gynecol 2010;116:1288–95.

20. Fang Y, Guirguis P, Borgida A, et al. Elective delivery with known fetal lung maturity prior to 39 wks is still associated with increased neonatal morbidity. Am J Obstet Gynecol 2011;204:S33–4.

21. Tita AT, Lai Y, Landon MB, et al; Eunice Kennedy Shriver National Institute of Child Health and Human Development (NICHD) Maternal-Fetal Medicine Units Network (MFMU). Timing of elective repeat cesarean delivery at term and maternal perioperative outcomes. Obstet Gynecol 2011;117:280–6.

22. Hutcheon JA, Lisonkova S, Joseph KS. Epidemiology of pre-eclampsia and the other hypertensive disorders of pregnancy. Best Pract Res Clin Obstet Gynaecol 2011;25: 391–403.

23. Smulian JC, Ananth CV, Vintzileos AM, et al. Fetal deaths in the United States. Influence of high-risk conditions and implications for management. Obstet Gynecol 2002;100:1183–9.

24. Spong CY, Mercer BM, D'alton M, et al. Timing of indicated late-preterm and early-term birth. Obstet Gynecol 2011;118:323–33.

25. Main EK. New perinatal quality measures from the National Quality Forum, the Joint Commission and the Leapfrog Group. Curr Opin Obstet Gynecol 2009;21:532–40.

26. Goldenberg RL, McClure EM, Bhattacharya A, et al. Women's perceptions regarding the safety of births at various gestational ages. Obstet Gynecol 2009;114:1254–8.

27. The Ohio Perinatal Quality Collaborative Writing Committee. A statewide initiative to reduce inappropriate scheduled births at 36(0/7)-38(6/7) weeks' gestation. Am J Obstet Gynecol 2010;202:243,e1–8. [Erratum in: Am J Obstet Gynecol 2010;202: 603].

28. Oshiro BT, Henry E, Wilson J, et al; Women and Newborn Clinical Integration Program. Decreasing elective deliveries before 39 weeks of gestation in an integrated health care system. Obstet Gynecol 2009;113:804–11.

29. Fisch JM, English D, Pedaline S, et al. Labor induction process improvement: a patient quality-of-care initiative. Obstet Gynecol 2009;113:797–803.

Index

Note: Page numbers of article titles are in **boldface** type.

Moving?

Make sure your subscription moves with you!

To notify us of your new address, find your **Clinics Account Number** (located on your mailing label above your name), and contact customer service at:

Email: journalscustomerservice-usa@elsevier.com

800-654-2452 (subscribers in the U.S. & Canada)
314-447-8871 (subscribers outside of the U.S. & Canada)

Fax number: 314-447-8029

**Elsevier Health Sciences Division
Subscription Customer Service
3251 Riverport Lane
Maryland Heights, MO 63043**

ELSEVIER

Printed and bound by CPI Group (UK) Ltd, Croydon, CR0 4YY

03/10/2024

01040456-0010